Community Care and Older People

Christina R. Victor
BA, M. Phil, Ph.D., Hon MFPHM
Department of Public Health Sciences
St George's Hospital Medical School
London

Stanley Thornes (Publishers) Ltd

First published 1997 by:
Stanley Thornes (Publishers) Ltd
Ellenborough House
Wellington Street
CHELTENHAM
GL50 1YW
United Kingdom

97 98 99 00 01 / 10 9 8 7 6 5 4 3 2 1

A catalogue record for this book is available from the British Library

ISBN 0-7487-3292-6

Cover photograph courtesy of Help the Aged

Typeset by Northern Phototypesetting Co Ltd., Bolton
Printed and bound in Great Britain by TJ International, Padstow, Cornwall

Dedication
For David and Christopher

Contents

Preface

Community care is a policy with few enemies. It is an objective upon which (almost) everyone can agree and as such appears uncontentious. Behind this mask of apparent dullness and uniformity there is a vibrant debate about what we mean by community care, how much we spend upon community care, and what the future of community care should be. In this book we look at these issues and how they affect older people who are in the main, passive recipients of these policies. There is a danger that we may take these vulnerable people as an experimental cohort for developing as yet unsubstantiated policy. Having written this book the author is aware that ideology and rhetoric have taken precedence over scientifically sound scholarship in informing policy developments.

The development of community care

INTRODUCTION

As far as older people are concerned 'the primary objective of departmental policies ... is to enable old people to maintain independent lives in the community for
as long as possible. To achieve this, high priority is being given to the development of domiciliary provision and the encouragement of measures designed to
prevent or postpone the need for long-term care in hospital or residential homes'
(DHSS, 1978, p. 13). Sentiments such as this, extolling the virtues of enabling
older people to continue to live independent lives, are not new. Means and Smith
(1985, p. 241) provide evidence from the annual reports of the Ministry of Health
(MoH) that such sentiments have been expressed over the last 40 years. For
example, in 1953 it was stated that there should be 'universal recognition of the
urgency of the task of enabling old people to go on living in their own homes as
long as possible'. In 1958 the report spoke of the emphasis being laid upon 'measures to enable elderly persons to remain in their own homes for as long as possible' and finally in 1960 'the general objective of both health and welfare
services, working in cooperation, is to maintain the elderly in the community and
to accept admission to hospital or residential care as the right course only where
an old person himself accepts the necessity for this and when he has reached a
point where community services are no longer sufficient'.

These diverse statements elegantly encapsulate the main features of the debate
about community care for older people which has characterized the post-war
period, especially avoiding the entry of older people into long-term care. This is
explicitly expressed as a 'bad thing' and something which both society and older
people themselves seek to avoid or at least avoid until as late as possible. However while there is an explicit reference to developing domiciliary provision there
is no explicit mention of the role of informal carers and the substituting of state
services with those provided by the wider community. However the debate has
broadened since 1953 and it is now argued that the care of elderly people is a res-

ponsibility which should be shared by all and is not one which is the exclusive pre-rogative of statutory services. Community care is the policy by which, it is hoped, this objective of helping older people to live independent lives within their homes for as long as possible can be achieved. In this book we look critically at the development and implementation of community care for older people from a population, or public health, perspective.

In this chapter we review the development of community care policy, with specific reference to older people in the UK in the period since 1945. However we concentrate upon the period leading up to the 1990 Community Care White Paper *Caring for People* (DoH, 1989). However it is important to remember that many of the issues noted in this chapter, such as the relationship between the formal and informal sectors, may also be observed throughout Europe and indeed further afield. Policy debates about community care and older people are therefore not confined to the UK but are also taking place in other countries (Scharf and Wenger, 1995; Challis *et al.*, 1994). In the final chapter of this book we will broaden our perspective and review the provision of community care for older people in Europe making direct comparisons with the situation in the UK where possible.

COMMUNITY CARE: THE ECONOMIC IMPERATIVE

As we shall see in a later section economic pressures have been an important stimulus in the development and implementation of community care for older people (and indeed other groups with long-term care needs). In this section we look at the overall expenditure upon community care as this provides the context within which to consider the development of this set of policies and the specific substantive topics examined in subsequent chapters (e.g. the role of the formal sector, long-stay care, the contribution of the informal sector).

It is easy to pose the question 'How much do we spend on community care? It is rather more difficult to provide a substantial answer as this depends upon the source and type of costing data used and assumptions about which services do (and do not) form part of community care. Furthermore it is often difficult to calculate costing data for specific client groups such as older people or those with learning difficulties.

Laing (1993) estimates the total expenditure on long-term care in the UK. He defines long-term care as continuing personal or nursing care for those unable to look after themselves; 'chronic' long-term patients who are not going to get 'better'. Using this definition such care may be provided in people's homes, day-centres or care home settings. He estimates an annual expenditure in 1992 on such care as £10.2 billion a year of which £9.1 billion is accounted for by elderly people. This accounts for 1.47% of the Gross Domestic Product (GDP). Of expenditure upon older people 70% comes from state sources and 30% from personal contributions. Long-stay care in institutional settings (e.g. nursing homes, residential homes) accounts for £6.6 billion a year (72.5% of the total long-term care expenditure on older people) and the state is responsible for 66% of this expenditure. However of the £2.5 billion spent upon providing services in older people's own homes 79% of this comes from the state. Hence older people (or their families) are much more likely to make a contribution to their long-term care in a residential/nursing home than for services received in their own home. This difference reflects the different ways in which these types of services have been organized and funded and is described in more detail later.

Robins and Wittenberg (1992) provide estimates of government expenditure upon different types of services such as health services, social services and social security payments for long- term care. In 1988/89 they estimate 51.9% of National Health Service (NHS) expenditure (this includes acute hospital care, long-term care and community health services such as community nurses and health services), 25% of Family Health Services (GPs, dentists, opticians) and 56.4% of expenditure on social services/social security long-term care payments were accounted for by older people. Overall older people accounted for 47% of the £11 350 million spent (although, of course, much of this is not community care as it includes the acute medical sector). Accepting the limitations of these data, Table 1.1 describes the estimated average per-capita expenditure on these services for older people. It is evident that average per-capita expenditure increases markedly with age and is approximately 4.5 times more for someone aged 85 years or more as compared with a person aged 65–74 years. These data combined with the ageing of the population are one of the most important reasons why the provision of health and social welfare services for older people has become a political issue and has been possibly the most important force in promoting interest in the broad policy objective of community care.

Table 1.1 Average per-capita expenditure (£) on health and social services for people aged 65+ (England 1989/90)[a]

Age (years)	Hospital and community health	Family health services	Personal social services	Income support for care	All
45–64	212	94	32	5	263
65–74	589	141	115	20	865
75–84	1195	214	333	125	1867[b]
85+	2193		1039	549	3995[b]
Total on elderly	7154	1303	2893		
% of all expended	51.9	25.0	56.4		

[a] Derived from Robins and Wittenberg, 1992, Tables 3.1 and 3.2
[b] Assumes family health expenditure of £214 applies to both 75–84 and 85+ age-groups

SETTING THE SCENE: THE CREATION OF THE WELFARE STATE

It is not the purpose of this book to provide a detailed description or analysis of the creation of the British welfare state. However to understand fully why the policy of community care developed and understand some of the current policy issues such as the debate about who pays for long-stay care, it is necessary to provide a very brief description of the creation of the welfare state. Further details concerning the development of social welfare in Britain are available elsewhere (Hills, 1993) as are detailed analyses of the development of welfare services for older people (Means and Smith, 1985; 1995).

The basic outline of the post-war British welfare state was outlined in the Beveridge Report published in 1942. This proposed the creation of a national health service and the development of a comprehensive social insurance system to cater for unemployment, sickness and old age. The report also suggested the replacement of all existing poor law legislation. The 1946 National Health Service Act resulted in the implementation of the National Health Service in July 1948. The founding principles of the NHS are:

- access to a comprehensive health care system is a 'right' of all citizens;
- access to health should be based on need and not the ability to pay;
- there should be both spatial and social equity of access to health care;
- health care services (including the 'hotel' element of in-patient care) are free at the point of consumption;
- the system is funded out of general taxation.

There are three very important features of the NHS which contrast with other types of social welfare. These are outlined below.

- Social and spatial equity of access to health care. This implies an aspiration towards a uniformity of provision and the notion of minimum levels of service. The emphasis was very much upon reducing variations in provision between areas.
- Health care was provided free at the point of consumption. Charges were not made for services, and access to services was not dependent upon 'means testing'.
- Health care was funded from general taxation.

Several aspects of the way the NHS was organized have effected the development of care for older people. Initially, the NHS was organized into three distinct components; the hospitals, the GPs (who remain independently contracted to the NHS rather than salaried employees) and the local health authorities who looked after community nursing and other community based health services. Although subject to considerable numbers of reorganizations since 1948, one constant theme has been the overwhelming power of the hospital sector within the NHS at the expense of other services. The provision of acute medical care in a hospital setting has always dominated the NHS. However the importance of the hospital medical sector has not been of particular benefit for the care and treatment of older people as 'medical staff from the hospital sector did not show equal enthusiasm for all types of patient; and, in particular, the treatment of elderly people was perceived as being of low status and priority' (Means and Smith, 1985, p. 127).

However, this bias against older people within the hospital sector was not a new feature associated with the creation of the NHS. It was observable in the hospital sector before the creation of the NHS and this was one of the major issues which resulted in the 1948 National Assistance Act. The voluntary, charitable and public health hospitals all concentrated upon the 'acute sick'. The 'chronic sick', a category within which mostly sick older people fell, were clustered in the hospitals still administered by public assistance committees (the successors of the poor law unions). The creation of the emergency medical service during the 1939–1945 period drew attention to the failure of the system to offer effective treatment to this group. The high numbers of beds occupied by older people was one important stimulus to the development of interest in the emerging specialty of geriatric medicine with its emphasis upon assessment and rehabilitation.

However, both central government and the medical profession assumed that it was possible to classify older people into a series of groups ranging from the well to those requiring constant care. In particular it was assumed that it was possible to differentiate between the acutely sick older people, the 'frail' who were in need of general attention and the 'chronic sick' who needed medical and nursing support. The NHS sought to concern itself with the first and third categories while the middle group were seen as being the responsibility of the the local authority via the creation of residential homes under the 1948 National Assistance Act. This has its modern parallel in that hospitals are increasingly concerning themselves with the acutely ill while local authorities have responsibility for social care needs.

In 1948 the National Assistance Act was passed. Under this legislation local authorities were given the power to provide residential homes to provide accommodation for those who were in need of care and attention. As noted above, one of the main concerns of social policy makers were the very large numbers of the 'chronic sick' elderly occupying hospital beds in public hospitals. Under this legislation local authorities were encouraged to reduce provision in the large general institutions and create specialist types of accommodation for different groups of people such as elderly people or those with learning disabilities.

Unlike the NHS, there was less concern for the ideal of equality of access to residential services. Instead, local authority services were enabled to respond flexibly to many of the responsibilities included within the 1948 act. Furthermore, local authority services were not provided free at the point of consumption. Those resident in such accommodation would be expected to pay for such care if they had the means. Hence, this type of care, unlike NHS health care, was not free at the point of consumption.

The National Assistance Act can be interpreted as an attempt to correct a very major issue of public concern. However, it did little to destroy the old 'workhouse' ethos because there was little consideration given to the staffing of these new homes. We will return to the debate about the role of residential care (Chapter 7). Outside the provision of residential care, local authorities were given few powers to provide services such as meals, clubs or chiropody, although they had very limited powers to make contributions to voluntary groups providing such services.

Why was such little attention given in the act to the development of domiciliary services for older people? Townsend (1981) argues that the emphasis upon residential care was a way of controlling older people by discouraging all but the most needy into its embrace. However Means and Smith (1985) consider that it reflects the narrow and unimaginative view of policy makers about the format of state sponsored social support for older people. It would appear that many individuals who were concerned with the development of policy in this area had little understanding of the reality of later life. They very readily accepted many rather negative stereotypes about the inability of older people to manage to live at home. Hence from their ideological perspective domiciliary services were seen as both unrealistic and inappropriate.

Early research studies into the lives of older people such as that of Sheldon (1948) in Wolverhampton, demonstrated the important role played by the family in the care of elderly people. However Means and Smith (1995) observe that such studies were published when there was concern that the creation of the 'welfare state' would encourage family members to reduce their responsibilities. They suggest that the reluctance to develop domiciliary based forms of provision was partly due to the fear that this would discourage informal care rather than promote and nurture it. It was only gradually that the latter argument gained acceptance.

THE DEVELOPMENT OF COMMUNITY CARE

With the implementation of the community care reforms in 1993 it is easy to assume that community care was 'invented' or 'created' in 1993. In fact this is a term that has been in use among policy makers for a considerable period. The precise origin of the term 'community care' remains obscure. Bulmer (1987) notes that the first official use of the term was in 1957 and related to the field of mental illness. However there has been a stream of community care related policy documents from central government over the last four decades (Table 1.2). Given the number of documents included within this list we will concentrate our attention upon the major reports and those with most impact.

The image of community care

In Britain, the development of community care policy during the late 1950s was fuelled by a reaction against the provision of care for the long-term chronically ill in communal or institutional settings, especially for those who were mentally ill. Institutions were perceived as inhumane, therapeutically ineffective and, perhaps most importantly of all, extremely expensive. As with many aspects of social welfare, concerns about the economic burden of providing care were starting to emerge alongside the development of a 'moral panic' (Jefferys, 1983). There were also concerns about the demographic trends in Britain, most specifically the 'ageing' of the population. Additionally, there was a gradual realization that providing domiciliary based services could encourage and promote family care and possibly prevent (or at least delay) admission to long-stay care.

Table 1.2 Community care: a chronology of policy development[a]

Date	Document
1957	Royal Commission on law relating to mental illness and mental deficiency
	Key point: first official use of term 'community care'
1963	Health and welfare: the development of community care
	Key point: promoted closure of institutions and replacement by community care
1973	NHS reorganization Act
	Key point: required health and local authorities to co–ordinate activities
1976	DHSS The way forward
	Key point: repeated commitment to community care
1978	A happier old age (DHSS/Welsh Office consultative paper)
	Key point: stressed role of voluntary and informal carers
1981	Growing older (White Paper)
	Key point: stressed care by the comunity
1985	House of Commons Social Services Committee report
1986	Audit Commission making a reality of community care
1987	Firth report on funding of residential care
	Key point: recommended common assessment policy for all types of homes
1988	Community Care : Agenda for Action (Griffiths report)
1989	White Papers: Caring for people/working for patients
1990	NHS and Community Care Act (NHSCCA): implemented in April 1991 NHS changes and 1993 community care changes

[a]After: Tinker *et al.* (1994)

In the field of long-stay care for older people, Townsend's book *The Last Refuge* (1964) carefully documented the appalling conditions which older people resident in these settings had to endure. Despite the rhetoric of the 1948 National Assistance Act, Townsend showed that relatively few 'new purpose' built residential homes had been constructed and that many older people remained in the former workhouses.

In contrast to the almost inevitable failings of long-stay provision, community care was seen as being both more effective and efficient as well as a more appropriate way of providing care for those who required support on a long term basis (see Means and Smith, 1995). Titmus (1968, p. 4) drew attention to the ideological nature of the word community as part of the term 'community care'. He used the powerful idealistic English image of the country cottage to evoke the warmth and positive nature of the term 'community'. He wrote 'What some hope will one

day exist is suddenly thought by many to exist already … what of the cottage gar-
den trailer "community care". Does it not conjure up a sense of warmth and human
kindness, essentially personal and comforting, as loving as the wild flowers so
enchantingly described by Lawrence in *Lady Chatterley's Lover*?' (Titmus, 1968,
p. 4). Communities are perceived as caring, integrated and harmonious entities
which existed in some previous 'golden age', (or other cultures), when older
people (or others with long-term care needs) were lovingly cared for by their kith
and kin and the community at large. This is contrasted, in popular imagery, with
the savage and inhumane regimes of institutional forms of provision and the fragmented, individualistic and uncaring nature of modern society.

These contrasting images hint at the types of characteristics which would typ-
ify the ideal or exemplary manifestation of community care policy. The ideal type
of community care model includes the following four core beliefs (Meredith,
1995):

- people prefer care at home (or in homely environments) to that provided in
  large institutional settings;
- institutions cannot by definition offer optimum personalized, individualist care
  or stimulating environments;
- each person requiring care must be treated with dignity and respect;
- the reorganization of services, agencies and ways of working will improve services and therefore the care received by individuals.

Howe describes the policy more cynically thus 'a ruse adopted by governments
is to champion the notion of community care. It sounds wholesome, it has that rosy
ring of nostalgia and yet it is an illusion' (Barrett, 1993, p. 13). While it is a point
of debate as to whether the entire concept of community care is an illusion, it is
beyond contention that the meaning behind this phrase has changed over time.
Over the past four decades, while the terminology has remained constant, the
meaning of the term 'community care' has undergone a subtle transformation.
This might appear, at first sight, to be no more than a simple academic exercise in
semantics. However, these changes have profoundly altered the reality of the policy and the types of support that older people (and other vulnerable groups) can
expect to receive. The multiple meanings and interpretations give the term 'community care' a lack of precision and clarity about which services should be provided and who should pay for them. This makes it possible for governments of all
political persuasions to argue in favour of this policy.

Care in the community and by the community

It is usual to distinguish between care in the community and care by the community.
Care in the community implies the use of statutory resources provided in clients' own
homes and in community based centres rather than the large impersonal institutions.
This manifestation of community care implies a significant input by state services.
Care by the community is associated with the mobilization of resources from within

the community such as voluntary organizations and informal carers such as friends, neighbours and kin. Thus, the main responsibility is seen as being taken by the community with statutory services being used only in extreme circumstances and as a last resort. This distinction was formally recognized by the government in the 1981 White Paper, *Growing Older*, with the statement that '... care in the community must increasingly mean care by the community' (DHSS, 1981a, p. 3).

This distinction between the forms of care implies two distinct models of community care. First, there is the notion of the community using its own resources to provide care through family and friends as well as voluntary and locally based formal services. Second, there is the idea that the communities resources will be supplemented by those from external sources e.g. national government. Increasingly in Britain, statutory services are seen as being used as the last resort in the care of older people; the care of older people is being placed firmly within the domain of the family and the informal sector. We will return to the issue of informal carers later in this book.

WHAT CONSTITITUTES COMMUNITY CARE?

As it is virtually impossible to be precise about the meaning of the term community care it is therefore difficult to be precise about what constitutes community care. The situation is made more complex because community care is a policy directive which is deemed appropriate for many different types of people (e.g older people, the mentally ill, people with HIV/AIDS). Consequently, the meaning and definition of community care may vary between groups. However, Meredith (1995) considers that community care would always include information, practical support (e.g. aids and adaptations), domestic assistance (to help with daily tasks), emotional support, physical/nursing care (to help with disability or illness), income maintenance, housing, transport and leisure and recreation.

In the broadest sense, community care includes at least four major dimensions; health care, social care, income maintenance and housing. However, a clear distinction has always been drawn in the minds of policy makers between health needs (the responsibility of the health sector) and those with social care needs (who, by and large, are the target group for community care). Operationalizing these definitions is not straightforward and the community care/health care relationship is littered with boundary disputes about the meanings of these terms.

Additionally, within these very broad areas of interest statutory agencies, voluntary agencies and private firms may be actively involved. In this book we are largely concerned with the social care aspects of community care and, to a lesser degree, how this relates to the health needs of older people. Where appropriate, the importance of income maintenance is noted as are aspects of housing policy. Constraints of space make it impossible to cover these two aspects in detail.

The essential elements of community care

Although the precise meaning of the term has altered over the years it remains possible to isolate several key features which are defining features of the general concept of community care. These may be summarized as:

- the provision of care outside large institutions such as hospitals or long-stay facilities;
- the provision of services and care outside the institutional setting and in the clients own home (or in as homely a setting as possible);
- the ideal of providing care in as normal, i.e. non-institutional setting as is possible given the needs of clients;
- a stress upon the involvement of members of the community in the care of those with long-term care needs;
- more recently a stress upon involving users and carers in the planning, development, delivery and monitoring of services.

However, as we have already indicated the balance between these different elements has varied over time and between the type of client group.

WHO PROVIDES COMMUNITY CARE?

We have already indicated that one of the distinguishing features of community care is the multiplicity of agencies involved in the implementation and delivery of services (irrespective of which statutory configuration of services we are considering). Community care is provided by both informal and formal providers. Formal providers are professional operators of services and consist of three main sectors; statutory agencies, the voluntary sector and the private sector. These are described briefly.

Statutory agencies

These are public bodies (such as local authorities or health authorities) who are established by law (or statute) and who are largely funded by the tax system.

Statutory provision for community care comes from two main sources; local authorities and health authorities. There are a variety of different levels (or tiers) of local authorities in the UK and some variation in structure between the constituent countries of the UK. Social services are provided by local authorities (such as counties like Surrey), London boroughs (like Merton), and the new unitary authorities. All these different types of local government are elected.

The structure of the health service now reflects the implementation of the 1991 changes (Baggott, 1994; Ham, 1992). These changes introduced the internal health market and separated out the role of health care purchasers (health authorities and GPs) from providers of services (health trusts such as St Georges Health

Care Trust). Purchasing authorities (the health commissions such as Kensington and Chelsea and Westminster Health Commission) are responsible for assessing the health care needs of their population and for purchasing appropriate health care. GPs who are fundholding (or involved in purchasing groups such as multi-funds) perform a similar function for their practice population. Neither of these agencies includes any elected representatives of the general population. Both sets of purchasers are involved in purchasing community care services. Health care services are provided by hospitals (which could be NHS trusts or private) and community health service trusts.

Voluntary sector agencies

These may provide particular services (e.g. the supply of Mobile Meals Services by the WRVS) or advance the cause of specific groups (e.g. Mencap, Mind or Age Concern). Voluntary agencies or charities receive funding from a variety of sources including donations from the public, grants from central/local government, sponsorship or charges for the services they provide. Typically the voluntary sector includes both paid and unpaid workers (volunteers) in their workforce, although just because a worker is a volunteer does not imply that they are untrained or inexperienced.

The private sector

As we will see, this is a major contributor to community care; mostly within the field of long-stay care (Chapter 7). Private sector firms undertake to provide certain services for an agreed fee but clearly they also need to be able to make a profit as a result of providing services. Given the myriad of agencies involved in the community care enterprise it is not surprising that the policy has been problematic.

THE DEVELOPMENT OF COMMUNITY CARE POLICY

Overall there has been a broad political and social consensus over the past 40 years about the appropriateness of community care as a social objective, especially for the care of older people. However, the policies have not been seen to be very effective. Consequently, the community care policy has been subject to recent rigorous scrutiny by a series of government reports; the Audit Commission (1986), the House of Commons Select Committee on Social Services (1985) and the Griffiths report (1986) which resulted in the 1989 White Paper *Caring for People* (DoH, 1989) and the 1990 NHS and Community Care Act (Table 1.2). These reports are briefly reviewed and the salient points highlighted. We then concentrate upon isolating the key issues which resulted in the NHS and Community Care Act (NHSCCA) and the eventual introduction of the community care legislation in

April 1993. Before moving on to a detailed review of these reports we briefly examine the initial impetus to the development of interest in community care.

Early pressure for reform: 1950–1980

As we have seen in the immediate postwar period (1945), public hospitals were the main method of providing care to those people with mental health problems and learning difficulties or those who were frail because of advanced age. It is as a result of concerns about the centrality of large hospitals in caring for this client group that there was the initial stimulus towards community care for *all* groups with long-term care needs (including the frail elderly).

What prompted the development of interest in the idea of community care so soon after the implementation of the welfare state? What brought about this policy change? Why did care in the large hospital setting become perceived as inappropriate? Why did community care become so popular with policy makers, politicians, lobby groups and lay people? There are no easy or simple answers to these questions. However, several factors would appear to be important; economic considerations (including population ageing); a concern with the quality of care offered; and a realization that there were possibilities for care outside institutional settings. These are considered below and will recur in our more detailed review of policy developments in the last decade.

One important stimulus towards reducing the provision of care in large hospitals was a longstanding concern about the high cost of such provision and the change in the demographic profile of the population. Concern about demographic trends; the declining birthrate and the ageing of the population, resulting in an increased demand for care, was an important stimulus to the development of community care. Indeed Means and Smith (1985) note that concerns about the changing demography of the UK have made health and social welfare provision important areas of political concern. The roots of this development may be seen in the early 1950s.

For people with learning disabilities or mental health problems powerful advocates such as MIND and Mencap started to question the pre-eminence of the institutional sector and argued for the development of community based forms of provision. A series of well publicized 'scandals' about the poor quality of care and ill treatment of patients in several long-stay hospitals for people with learning disabilities (e.g. Ely and South Ockendon) raised questions about the basic levels of care experienced by all clients in the long-stay hospital sector.

Powerful stereotypes and very negative images of older people (and probably those with mental health problems or learning disabilities) were prevalent and doubts about their abilities to live in non-institutional settings. For example, Means and Smith (1985) note that it was commonly assumed that frail older people could not live on their own, however much the older person might want to. The prevailing assumption was that such people were much better off in an institutional environment.

Early progress towards community care

In response to extensive media concern about the quality of care experienced by those still resident in long-stay hospitals, two White Papers were issued in 1971 *Better services for the mentally handicapped*) and 1977 (*Better services for the mentally ill*). Although not explicitly concerned with older people, both these documents argued against the large long-stay hospitals and for their replacement with community based services. Despite the production of a consultative document in 1981: *Care in the community* (DHSS, 1981b); and a subsequent circular (DHSS, 1983) progress towards the stated policy goal of running down long-stay provision and its substitution by enhanced community services was extremely slow.

One reason for the slowness of the development of community care was the fragmented way that services were provided. As a result of the division of responsibilities between agencies for the provision of primary care, health and social services clearly did not help expedite the move towards community care regardless of client group. Indeed a major reason articulated for many of the reforms of the NHS and social service systems in the UK has been the goal of improving the coordination of care between different parts of the health and social care system (Ham, 1992; Baggott, 1994).

Developments in the 1980s

In the mid 1980s there was another renewed and more general interest expressed in the move towards community care. Again, it is difficult to identify precisely what stimulated this interest. However it seems to stem from two interrelated factors; concerns about the ageing of the population and the growth of public sector funding of private sector residential and nursing homes. The concern about demographic change and the ageing of the population was not new. Neither were the high service utilization rates of the over 75s new. However these issues seem to have been rediscovered, and the impact of demographic change upon the health and welfare services became an issue of major political significance in a way that had not been true in the first decade of the welfare state (DHSS 1981a).

There was a new stimulus towards the development of community care and this was the growth of private residential and nursing homes. In the early 1980s, there was a minor change in the claiming of supplementary benefit (supplementary pension for older people) – both benefits were subsequently replaced by income support. The change made it possible for older people on low incomes, who were entitled to supplementary pension, to enter private nursing or residential homes and to have their fees paid by the social security system. Under these circumstances, entry to the private care sector was based upon demonstration of financial entitlement rather than upon any 'objective' assessments of the older persons need for care.

As a consequence of this change there was a huge growth in the number of private homes, the number of places provided by such homes and a massive increase in the amount of money being spent by the social security system on maintaining mainly older people in private care homes (although some of the expenditure did go on people with learning disabilities). We will look in detail at the changes in the provision of long-stay care for older people in Chapter 7. However, to demonstrate the scale of the impact this rather minor change in the supplementary benefit regulation had upon the system, the number of places provided by the private sector increased from 46 900 (1982) to 161 200 in 1991 (an increase of 340%) (Laing, 1993); expenditure increased from £10 (1979) to £1872 per annum in 1991 (Laing, 1993) and the number of people receiving such payments increased from 12 000 (1979) to 90 000 (1986) (Means and Smith, 1995).

Community care in the 1980s: The emergence of critical reports

Major policy reports on community care will now be considered. The reports discussed below are important milestones towards the implementation of the community care reforms in 1993. The significance and impact of especially the House of Commons and Audit Commission reports is attributable to several factors. These include the independent, impartial views of the reports' authors, and the way in which they collected and analysed pertinent information.

House of Commons Social Services Committee Report 1985

Although this report was concerned with the community care of adults with mental health problems or learning disabilities, the concerns and issues raised are relevant to those of older people. The main issues raised in this report are outlined below.

- Policy was biased towards getting people out of hospitals. There was an assumption that hospitals were no longer required when caring for those with long term care problems.
- Most people with long-term care needs were already being cared for in the community (mainly by their family). This fact needed to be acknowledged in the development of policy. We will return to this point in chapter six.
- There was no agreement on either the definition of 'community care' or on what constituted 'good' community care.
- The run down of the network of large hospitals was proceeding faster than the development of replacement community based services.
- There was no appropriate financial mechanism for achieving the stated policy objective.
- Joint planning mechanisms obviously needed strengthening and, very importantly, the views of users and carers needed to be listened to, especially in the development of services.

The official response to this report was negligible, although Means and Smith (1995, p. 51) note that it was conceded that 'a good community based service was likely to be more expensive than a bad hospital service'. Such candidness has not been repeated, and it has been widely assumed that community care will be cheaper than institutional or collective forms of provision.

The Audit Commission Report 1986

The Audit Commission Report *Making a reality of community care* was published in 1986. Its focus was upon the movement of those with long-term care problems (mental health, learning disabilities and frail elderly) from hospitals to community services. This report re-evaluated the whole policy of community care and concluded that the policy was a failure and that this failure was not the result of local level planning failures but of central government policy itself. The report noted that when people had been moved out of large institutions they had often been relocated into smaller ones such as nursing homes rather than genuine community based services. More specifically the report identified key issues.

- The multiplicity of funding sources for community care. Funds for community care developments derived from various sources (e.g. NHS, local authority). These were often not coordinated and the mechanisms for allocating and distributing funds failed to take into account the changing responsibilities of the agencies involved (e.g. the transfer of responsibilities from NHS to local authority social service departments).
- The lack of 'bridging' funds to facilitate the switch from hospital to community based forms of provision.
- The 'perverse' financial incentive generated by the social security system. This highlighted the point noted earlier that the social security system was being used to provide care in institutional settings. However, no funds were available if people wished to remain in their own homes. This was quite clearly in total opposition to all stated policy objectives.
- The organizational failings that existed. Numerous agencies were involved in the development of community care. Given the structure of the NHS and local authorities at the time, there was confusion as to where the responsibilities for developing and managing the policy actually lay. There was no systematic approach to the formulation of care arrangements and the costing of different plans.

The damning nature of the report and its warnings of dire consequences of failure to act persuaded the government of the day to accept the report's suggestion that a high level review be initiated. Consequently, the then Secretary of State, Norman Fowler, invited Sir Roy Griffiths to undertake a review of community care.

The Griffiths Report

The remit of this report was 'to review the way public funds are used to support community care policy and to advise [the Secretary of State] on the options for action which would improve the use of these funds as a contribution to more effective community care.' Underlying the review were key themes:

- that adequate resources were required;
- that government must take community care more seriously;
- that current problems resulted from a policy failure at a national (not local) level;
- that responsibilities were unclear and coordination inadequate;
- that the role of the social security system in subsidizing community care was wasteful;
- that choice and efficiency would be promoted by the development of a mixed economy of care (ie competition between private, public and voluntary sector providers). This main points from this report are described below. They are presented in some detail so that the original recommendations may be compared with what was eventually included within the 1991 NHS and Community Care Act.

The Griffiths Report stressed three key policy objectives:

- the promotion of non-institutional forms of care which would enable people to remain in their own home;
- the centrality of the services user (and their carer) by identifying and meeting needs and promoting choice;
- the targeting of services and resources for those 'most in need' and the avoidance of duplication and waste.

A series of proposals and recommendations were included in this report. The main points raised in the report were as outlined below.

- It was suggested that there should be the appointment of a Minister of Community Care who would provide a strategic overview and ensure progress towards the specified policy objectives. Earmarked community care funds would be made available to local authority social services departments.
- It was proposed that social services should become the lead agency in community care with responsibilities for *all* client groups. Identification of need, the creation of 'packages of care' and coordination of care were to be their main functions as well as regulation of nursing/residential homes.
- This changed role of the local authority was emphasized in that they were to be enabling agencies, not monopolistic providers of care as had previously been the case and that a mixed economy of care be developed.
- Another recommendation was that housing authorities were to confine themselves to the 'bricks and mortar' aspect of community care.
- Health authorities, it was suggested, should retain responsibilities for 'health' needs and would be required to provide the necessary inputs into assessing needs and care packages.
- Entry to publicly funded nursing and residential care should be through a rigorous assessment of needs for care and financial need.

● Targeting of resources would be a 'fact of life' and, in future, public subsidy would be aimed at those on low income. Those in less modest circumstances were to be expected to plan for their 'old age'.

A number of criticisms may be levelled at The Griffiths Report. First it made rather sweeping assumptions about the financial circumstances of current (and future) generations of elderly people which are not supported by research evidence (Falkingham and Victor, 1991). Second, while the report officially recognized the previously invisible army of informal carers and their role in caring for elderly people in the community it did not acknowledge the burdens and psychological problems generated. Third, the role of housing in developing community care was almost totally ignored. Fourth, the development of the mixed economy of care, largely by the creation of an enhanced private sector in the delivery of domiciliary care was treated as entirely unproblematic. Finally, it was assumed that it was possible to divide those who required 'social care' from those with health care needs. This division of responsibilities between agencies was treated as entirely unproblematic.

The Community Care White Paper

The Griffiths Report was published in March 1988 but the White Paper on community care, *Caring for People* (DoH, 1989) was not published until November 1989. This delay is widely thought to have occurred because several of the Griffiths' recommendations did not fit easily with the anti-local authority ideology of the government. Ultimately, the White Paper reflected many of the recommendations included in The Griffiths Report (probably because almost every other option was deemed unworkable).

Caring for People is based upon the assumption that for most people community care is the 'best' form of care available. The ideology underpinning this report, therefore, promotes the ideals of the family as the main source of care and the home as the appropriate place to receive such care. The White Paper states that the proposed changes are intended to:

● enable people to live as normal a life as possible in their own homes or in a homely environment in the community;'
● provide the right amount of care and support to enable people to achieve maximum independence;
● provide people with a greater say in how they live their lives and the services they need.

The White Paper identifies the key components of community care as services which:

● respond sensitively and flexibly to the needs of individuals and their carers;
● allow a range of options for consumers;
● do not intervene more than is necessary to promote independence;

• concentrate upon those with the greatest needs.

The White Paper states six main objectives for service delivery in the field of community care. These are noted below along with some of the major implicit issues.

Domiciliary, day and respite services

The first objective was to promote the development of domiciliary, day and respite services to enable people to live in their own homes and to target these at those 'most in need'.

This objective covers three types of services; domiciliary, day and respite. Domiciliary services are those actually received in an elderly person's home such as home help services or mobile meals services. Day services are those provided outside a person's actual home such as day centres or day hospitals. Respite care refers to services provided to allow regular carers a break (or respite) from their task. Again, this can take several forms ranging from someone looking after the dependent while the carer goes out, to admission of the dependent to hospital or other facility while the carer has a holiday.

Central to this objective is the notion of targeting resources at those most 'in need'. A perceived failure of social services prior to the introduction of the community care reforms was that services were spread too 'thinly' and did not concentrate upon those with the greatest needs. However the 'preventative' contribution such apparently small scale interventions could make was not recognized.

Support for informal carers

Another objective was to ensure that services providers made support for informal carers a high priority. The White Paper represents the first official acknowledgement of the extensive role played by the informal sector in the care of older people (and others with long-term care needs). While the importance of carers was acknowledged they were not initially seen as important in their own right. Only with the introduction of an amendment to the NHS and Community Care Act, which came into effect in April 1996, did carers become eligible for an assessment of their needs (although this does not entitle them to any services).

Need and good case management: assessment

It was stated that there should be proper assessment of need and good case management and that this should be the key to the provision of good quality care. The resultant care packages should reflect individual needs and preferences.

As we have seen, a major stimulus towards the development of the community care reforms was the large amount of money spent on residential and nursing home care without individuals undergoing any form of 'rigorous' assessment as to whether they needed such forms of care. When there was assessment this was often undertaken by a multiplicity of health and social care professionals in total isolation from one another. Consequently an elderly person who needed help around the home, help with personal care and some aids or adaptations provided could find herself being assessed three times (by the home care organizer for home help, by the district nurse for help with bathing and by the occupational therapist for aids/adaptations). A key feature of the new system is that such unnecessary duplication was reduced and that complex assessments would be coordinated by the local authority.

Furthermore, there had been a widespread unease that decisions about the services provided for elderly people were made on the basis of what was available rather than what was actually needed by the individual. For example, an individual might be offered help with home care when what was really required was help in cutting the hedge.

The development of private, public and voluntary sector cooperation

It was suggested that it was necessary to promote the development of the independent sector working alongside the public and voluntary sector and to 'refocus' the role of local authorities towards becoming enabling (or purchasing) agencies rather than direct providers of care. It is part of the underlying philosophy of the Conservative administration which introduced these reforms, that by developing markets in social care (and indeed education and health) the competition between providers will increase the choice and quality of services offered while reducing costs. The development of the mixed economy of care is one of the central planks of the reforms and success in achieving this objective is critical.

The accountability of agencies

It was felt that it was necessary to clarify the responsibilities of agencies to increase accountability. Another key element of the reforms was the issue of accountability. The identification of elected local authorities as the lead agency for the implementation and management of community care was one example of the reforms thrust towards clearly identified responsibilities. Another manifestation of this aim was that the act intended that users and carers would know who provided which services and how these could be accessed.

One important area of confusion is, however, the demarcation between health and social care for those with long-term care needs. While the White Paper very clearly stated that the responsibilities for health authorities remained the same, local authorities took over responsibility for assessing those who wished to enter publicly funded nursing care. As we shall see in Chapter 7, this had led to considerable confusion as to where the responsibility for providing long-term care for some client groups actually rests.

To secure 'better value for money'

This objective reflects again the generally ideological stance of the government that introduced these changes. Indeed, a similar objective was stated for the introduction of the NHS changes. However, with regard to community care, this again highlights the perverse financial incentive to place people in residential/nursing homes which had existed before.

The key recommendations of this White Paper are summarized briefly as:

- local authorities should be the lead agency in developing community care with the responsibility to assess the needs of individuals for care and develop an appropriate package of services within the resources available;
- the requirement for local authorities to publish clear plans for the development of community care services;
- the development of a mixed economy of welfare provision, using the private, voluntary and public sectors. The local authority will be expected to make maximum use of the private sector. Consequently the local authority should become an enabling authority rather than a monopolistic provider of care. There is to be a split between those parts of the local authority who directly provide care for clients (providing agencies) and those who purchase care for clients (purchasing authorities);
- local authorities to be responsible for the provision of social care while medical care remains the province of the NHS;
- the institution of new funding arrangements from April 1991. This will mean that local authorities will manage a social care budget regardless of whether the care is provided at home or in an institution;
- there should be a single method of entry for those being supported by public funds irrespective of the type of institution (i.e. public, private, voluntary) which they wish to enter. The local authority will take over financial responsibility for the support of new applicants for such care;
- further, the distinction between sectors in terms of standards and regulatory procedures would be abolished with a single set of standards for all residential facilities.

The White Paper goes into some detail as to how these objectives should be achieved, but it is beyond the scope of this volume to describe these in detail. However, it is worth indicating that the paper does set specific priorities for 'elderly and disabled people'. This heading, which the report uses, is illuminating as it indicates that, for the government, old age and disability are synonymous. The priorities set are as follows:

- the promotion of positive lifestyles through health education, health surveillance, and screening to reduce the need for in-patient and residential care;
- the promotion of coherent networks of services which assist people to live dignified and independent lives in the community;
- the provision of a full range of services;

- the avoidance of unnecessary institutional care by assessment of needs for care;
- improved access to information about services at both local and national services.

For older people in particular, the White Paper is full of references to the need to avoid unnecessary admission to institutions. In the government's mind this is obviously an extensive problem, but no evidence is given as to the number of older people to whom this happens.

According to Hunter and Judge (1988), there are three main general policy objectives which are enshrined in the report. First, there is a generalized concern about the need to ensure that appropriate services are provided for those who need them i.e. a concern with the effective targeting of resources to those deemed 'most in need'. Second, there is the imperative to take into account seriously the views of those using services and to provide them with greater choice. Third, there is the requirement to provide care in their own homes, whenever possible, with a stress upon providing care in as normal a setting as is possible given the clients needs. Hence the review is very clear that 'the family' or a family type of environment is the best way of meeting the needs of individuals.

These changes pointed to a fundamental change in the role and function of local authorities. The three key tasks which they were to undertake in their new role were outlined.

- There should be the assessment of an individual's need for *social* care (including residential and nursing homes) in collaboration with other relevant agencies before deciding which services should be provided. Hence, social services departments were to move from a service-led system of service delivery to a needs-led service.
- After assessment, packages of care designed to meet the identified individual needs should be designed. Case managers (later care managers) were to be the organizers of these packages.
- They should stop acting as direct monopolistic providers of care and develop their purchasing and contracting role and become enabling authorities (rather similar to health authorities). As well as assessing individual needs, local authorities were to develop their macro level of strategic role of need assessment through the development of community care plans.

Not all the recommendations of the Griffiths review were, however, included in the White Paper. No Minister for Community Care was appointed and there was no system of 'earmarked' funds. However, the White Paper introduced a complaints procedure and proposed a system of inspection for residential care in all sectors.

A new funding structure for those people being funded by the state and who wished to enter residential care was prepared. Local authorities were to take over responsibility for the financial support of people in private and voluntary homes over and above their entitlement to social security. This was to be funded by a transfer of money from the social security budget to local authorities who would then have discretion over how much of this money would be spent on residential care (and how much of this should be spent on developing community based services).

CONCLUSION

Before considering the current organizational arrangements for the provision of community care it is instructive to try to draw together the common themes which have run through the practice of community care over the last decades. There has been concern with the 'cost' of different forms of care and demographic change, conflicts in the allocation of service priorities, conflicts between agencies, and changes in the philosophy underpinning the provision of welfare services.

At the heart of the debates about community care has been a continued concern with the 'cost' of providing services to an increasingly ageing population which has a deceasing percentage of its population gainfully employed. This concern was important in stimulating the interest in the development of community based alternatives. When such services are based upon the provision of care through the formal sector, the issue of cost is again raised as the 1986 Audit Commission report acknowledge. Hence the concern about cost has increasingly led to a retrenchment of statutory agencies and the increased emphasis placed upon the role of the informal sector.

A further and, as yet, largely unresolved issue, which inhibits the development of community care, relates to the issues of 'priorities' for funding. This has two dimensions; the difficulty in establishing the care of the chronically ill as a priority for funding and the competition between different priority groups for funding. Despite nearly 50 years of the NHS, the acute hospital sector still has pre-eminence in competitions for funding and the allocation of resources. As in 1946 the care of the chronically ill/frail older person remains very low down on the list of funding priorities. Older people and other community care recipient groups remain the 'Cinderella' care groups.

Conflicts between the agencies and professional groups involved in the development and implementation of community care are a constant feature of the last 50 years. For a variety of reasons multiprofessional working remains highly problematic. Furthermore there is a continuing conflict between central and local agencies about how community care is organized. The philosophy of community care incudes the belief that services are most appropriately planned and provided at the local level. This devolution of power to the local level does not rest comfortably with the overriding desire of governments to contain (or reduce) public expenditure.

Philosophical changes in the nature of the welfare state have taken place and this has influenced the way we think about community care. Three main changes characterize the last 50 years. First, there is the move from universal provision (where provision is available to all on the basis of need) to selective (or targeted) provision (where access to provision is dependent upon the means of the individual and is restricted to those in 'greatest need'). Second, is the move from a situation where care was provided almost exclusively by the public sector to a 'mixed' economy of provision (i.e. the development of welfare markets involving public, voluntary agencies and private sector as care providers). Third, is the move from the notion of collective (or state) provision to a situation where individuals are increasingly expected to provide for themselves with the state assuming responsibility for a decreasing percentage of the population. These changes have implications for older people as they are the prime users of state provided welfare services. In the next chapter we will look at how community care has been implemented.

2 | Organization and implementation of community care

INTRODUCTION

The new arrangements for community care were included in the National Health Service and Community Care Act (NHSCCA) which was passed in June 1990. The health service changes were implemented in April 1991. However, implementation of the community care component of the legislation was phased in over a two year period (April 1991 – April 1993). In this section we will confine our attention to the effect the new legislation has had upon the way social service departments are organized and how this differs from previous arrangements.

Included in the NHSCCA were objectives to be achieved by community care as well as organizational arrangements by which these would be achieved. As Hughes (1995) observes it was through these organizational changes that central government further sought to promote its basic policy of marketing public sector services. The main organizational changes were as outlined below.

- As with health care the social care sector was to be separated into purchasers of care and providers of care. This separation of purchaser–provider functions was seen as the mechanism by which a market in social care could be created. The creation of such a market would result in competition between providers for contracts resulting in improved efficiency and increased quality of services.
- The delivery of services to both users and carers was to be achieved through a comprehensive system of assessment and care management. People would not be expected to fit services, rather their needs were to be assessed and a tailored package of care delivered.
- Social service departments had to demonstrate that the planning of services and outcomes had been achieved by working collaboratively with various interested agencies such as health authorities, voluntary agencies and user/carer groups.

These changes resulted in a fundamental restructuring of the way social service departments are now organized. Prior to the introduction of the NHSCCA, the 'typical' social service department was organized in one of two main ways; by function or by client group. For example, a functionally organized social service department might have been divided into three main groups; fieldwork, residential services and administration – while a client based set of organizational arrangements might have seen a department divided into three service based groups; children and families, adults and elderly people.

Following the implementation of the NHSCCA, these types of internal organization are no longer appropriate. Consequently social service departments tend to be organized around the four main tasks that they have to achieve in order to implement the community care legislation. These are assessment, care management, commissioning and quality assurance. Each of these areas of responsibility are reviewed in turn. Some of these issues will also feature in later chapters.

ASSESSMENT

Assessment of need is, in theory at least, the centrepiece of community care. The White Paper very clearly laid down the duty of the local authority to assess people needing 'social care and support – e.g. for mobility, personal care, domestic tasks ...' (DoH, 1989, para. 3.2.2). These assessments should 'take account of the wishes of the individual and his or her carer ... efforts should be made to offer flexible services which enable individuals and carers to make choices' (DoH, 1989, para. 3.2.6). These assessments should not focus upon the eligibility of individuals for particular services but are intended to identify a comprehensive picture of an individual's needs. These assessments of need are therefore individually based, and will be examined further (Chapter 4).

The local authority is also responsible for needs assessment at the population or macro level in order to develop their community care plans. One approach to this population level needs assessment is to combine (or aggregate) the information collected from the individual assessments. However to achieve this requires a standardized method of undertaking the individual assessments and then a method for aggregating the information. In this section we are examining the principles and legislative basis for these activities. We will examine the methodological and substantive aspects of population and individually based needs assessment for community care in Chapters 3 and 4 respectively.

Population level assessment of needs for community care

At a population level (which could be a locality, borough or county) the local authority has to collect, collate and interpret relevant data to enable it to produce an annual community care plan. This plan must state the objectives and priorities for community care and set targets for achieving these. Community care plans are public documents and must link with the plans of other relevant agencies such as housing or health.

In Chapter 3 we will look at the detailed requirements which community care plans are required to fulfil, as this provides the framework or context for the population level needs assessment. A major theme inherent in the community care legislation in general and community care plans in particular is the issue of consultation with users, carers and relevant local organizations as well as other relevant agencies such as housing and health. This relates back to one of the key themes in the original Griffiths report; the empowerment of users and carers.

What is meant by 'consultation'? Clearly there are a variety of frameworks of involvement which would enable the local authority to meet the government's requirement for the involvement of users and carers. It is useful to distinguish between two distinct paradigms of involvement (although in the 'real world' this is clearly a continuum of involvement). At one extreme there is the model of involvement in which users and carers are shown a plan, after it has been developed but prior to publication, and they are invited to 'comment' upon its content. We may contrast this with the other extreme of involvement when the planning process actually involves all relevant parties.

The extent and models of users and carers involvement in the community care planning process remains unclear, mainly because the legislative changes were made fairly recently. Means and Smith (1995) indicate that while most community care plans show evidence of extensive consultation with health and voluntary agencies there is, as yet, little evidence of the active involvement of users and carers in this process. Glendenning and Bewley (1992) support this conclusion by reporting that, of the 99 community care plans they studied, only 16% clearly stated the involvement of users and carers.

Given the newness of this task, it is not surprising that local authorities are still trying to define effective ways of involving users and carers in the planning process. However involving users, carers and local organizations in the community care planning process is not as straightforward as it might appear at first sight. Meredith (1995) documents the types of 'hard to reach' groups which must be involved if consultation in community care is not to become just a token 'paper' exercise. These groups include those who are not current users but who might become so in the future, the housebound, the visually impaired/deaf, those who do not speak/understand English, those who are unfamiliar with the language of social services and those with transport difficulties.

Means and Smith (1995) suggest that, in order to promote the active involvement of users and carers, a variety of issues need to be addressed. These are:

- the accessibility of attending meetings (this includes the physical accessibility of the buildings used and the ability of users/carers to attend them e.g. the need to cover the costs of looking after a dependent to facilitate a carer attending a meeting);
- the availability of appropriate information to all relevant parties;
- clarity about the degree of influence that users/carers will be able to exert;
- advocacy and support for those who are not used to being asked for their views

in order that their voices may be heard effectively;

- sufficient time for the consultation process so that the process does not become one of simple ratification;
- ensure that users/cares receive feedback on the results of the consultation process highlighting areas where they have (and have not) influenced the planning process;
- administrative and decision-making structures within authorities should be developed which allow the input of the views of users and carers.

Involving other agencies: the health–social care divide

Community care is concerned with the provision of social care while health authorities are concerned with health care. This begs the question; 'what are 'health care' and 'social care'? Despite early attempts to define these concepts there is no national definition of these two concepts. Instead, it is stated that 'The government has not thought it appropriate to attempt to define a rigid demarcation between health and social care; the interface between the two is for local discussion and agreement'. (DoH, 1991b, para. 4.20).

However, distinguishing between these two concepts has, in practice, been difficult as reported by the Association of Directors of Social Services (ADSS, 1994). In the past 'health workers' have undertaken social care tasks and vice versa. However social care services, such as cleaning, shopping or the provision of meals, are often seen as being provided by untrained, 'non-professional' staff. In contrast health services are provided by trained and professional staff. However blurring the boundaries between these two types of care is one mechanism by which 'seamless' provision of care can be achieved.

One example of the boundary disputes which can cause confusion in the implementation of community care is bathing services. Few would take issue with the premise that personal cleanliness is a fundamental requirement. However there are often disputes between health and social care agencies as to whether bathing is a social or health care responsibility. As Ebrahim (1994, p. 298) states 'a social bath is a bath that anyone can do but no-one will pay for'.

However Means and Smith (1995) conclude that there has been much greater progress in involving health authorities in community care planning than users or carers. They consider that, where local authority and health authority boundaries are contiguous good progress can emerge. They use the 1992–93 community care plan from St Helens as an example of what can be achieved. This plan includes agreed definitions of social care and health care and then applies these definitions to a range of 150 different tasks. In this area social care is defined as interventions designed to address the following needs:

- practical assistance with daily living (e.g. provision of food, and assistance with personal care);
- practical advice and help in coping with day to day problems;
- specific teaching and guidance to acquire new skills or reinforce existing ones

(e.g. preparing young people to leave care);
- specialized programmes of care assessment, treatment and rehabilitation which aim to improve the function of individuals so that they may live more freely and independently;
- protecting children at risk.

Table 2.1 The division of tasks between health and social care agencies[a]

Task	Responsibility
a) DoH	
Home management	social care
Laundry	social care
Incontinence laundry	either health or social care agency
Management of incontinence	health care
Washing/dressing	either
Bathing	either
Injections	health care
b) St Helens	
12 House care tasks	social care
3 Food preparation tasks	social care
Feeding	either/both agencies
6 Self-care tasks	either or both

[a]Derived from Ebrahim, 1994, Table 1; Means and Smith, 1995, Table 6.1

How does this affect the specific tasks with which older people might need help? This framework was then applied to a variety of different tasks a sample of which are shown in Table 2.1. Most of the domestic care tasks were seen as 'social care' (e.g. house care tasks) and none as health care; all 11 personal care tasks were seen as being the responsibility of both or either authority with none being seen as the sole responsibility of the social care agencies (Means and Smith, 1995). A similar division of responsibility was suggested by the Department of Health (DoH, SSI, 1991b) (Table 2.1). In both cases, a large number of tasks are seen as being the responsibility of either authority. The danger here is not that there will be duplication of effort but rather that neither will provide these services. It remains unclear as to how such guidelines are being utilized on the ground. Clearly such guidance is only a start and one would seek deeper cooperation in the future, perhaps resulting in joint commissioning of services as suggested by Henwood et al. (1991).

In the interim period, while there is a lack of agreed definition about which facilities should be provided and by whom, there will be considerable variations across the country in the type of services available to older people. Further this variation in the division of responsibility means that some older people will be contributing towards the services they receive, because they are being provided by a social care agency, while others will not because the same services are being provided by the health care sector.

Targeting and priorities

To aim towards and establish priorities for community care plans it is necessary for local authorities to set targets for services. These two related objectives mirror the requirements of health authorities to undertake similar activities. In the health field this has resulted in a debate about which services should and which should not be funded by the health services. In the social care service, targets should be measurable rather than vague assertions (e.g. the provision of a specified number of day care places or achieving a certain level of staffing). However the setting of targets alone does not ensure that a high quality service is provided. Furthermore, by setting priorities for service provision, some people with identified needs might not have these needs met because they do not fall into the priority groups identified.

Individual assessments

We will consider the detail of the assessment of individual needs in Chapter 4. Perhaps the defining principle of the community care changes was the notion that publicly funded social care services were provided on the basis of the assessment of the individuals need for care. Under the NHS and Community Care Act, assessment of need for community care services became a duty of the local authority. The local authority is expected to assess all those needing 'social care and support – e.g. for mobility, personal care, domestic tasks, financial affairs, accommodation, leisure and employment, which they cannot arrange for themselves' (DoH, 1989, para. 3.2.2). The 'assessment should take account of the wishes of the individual and his or her carer, and of the carer's ability to continue to provide care. Efforts should be made to offer flexible services which enable individuals and carers to make choices' (DoH, 1989, para. 3.2.6).

However, it is important to remember that assessment does not imply entitlement for services or that such services will be provided. In putting this duty into operation the local authority has to set out the conditions under which assessments of need will take place. These include; who is eligible for assessment, how to apply for assessments, what format will the assessment take and how can users/carers make representations and complaints about the assessment process. We will return to these points and many of the dilemmas concerning the assessment process in Chapter 4. Again, it is important to note that each local authority has its own system for the implementation of the assessment system. Consequently older people living in different parts of the country will be covered by different assessment and eligibility criteria.

CARE MANAGEMENT

The Department of Health (DoH/SSI, 1991a) consider that there are three stages to the comprehensive care management process. These stages are:

- assessment of the users' circumstances;
- the development of an agreed care package to meet identified need within existing resources;
- the implementation and monitoring of the package.

Consequently, care management relates to the process by which an agreed package of care, generated by the assessment process, is implemented and monitored. A care plan should include objectives for the provision of services. These objectives (e.g. keeping an older person at home and out of institutional care) should be agreed with users and carers.

The care plan and care management part of the community care process takes place in a financial context; care managers operate within the framework of available resources. In some authorities care managers are responsible for the budgets while in others this responsibility lies with other groups in the authority. Again, diversity in the organization of the care management process is a key feature of the implementation of community care. Care managers (it was originally referred to as care management) must also continue to monitor the changing needs of individuals.

We have already noted that the previous system of social care was thought to be flawed because people were fitted into the existing services provided rather than services being provided which met their requirements for help. The government felt that such inadequacies could be overcome by the needs-led assessment process and the care management approach. Six major objectives were identified for care management:

- ensuring that available resources are used in the most effective way to meet identified individual needs;
- promoting independence by enabling people to live in the community;
- preventing/minimizing the effects of illness and disability;
- treating those who need services with dignity and respect and providing equal opportunities for all;
- promoting individual choice and self-determination;
- promoting partnership between users, carers and services providers (from all sectors).

Progress towards the development of care management

In order to understand the problems local authorities are having in moving towards care management, it is necessary to understand the development of this approach. Care management emerged from North America as a way of navigating older people through the numerous health and welfare agencies involved in their care. In this setting the care manager was not a service provider but a broker or advocate.

In the UK, the care management projects in Thanet and Gateshead (Challis and Davies, 1986) proved very influential in stimulating interest in the approach.

These projects reported that older people who had experienced the care management scheme were less likely to die prematurely and less likely to enter long-term care than their contemporaries while their carers felt more supported. However, there are difficulties with these projects (Fisher, 1990; Means and Smith, 1995), which are acknowledged by the research team, but which make implementing care management by local authorities problematic. First, the older people who were chosen to participate in the research were very carefully selected which, of course, limits the impartiality of the study. Second, the positive results demonstrated apply to a limited group of frail elderly people. Therefore, it is not clear if such benefits would apply to other groups, such as the mentally ill or those with learning disabilities.

As there is more than one style of care management and a multiplicity of approaches this creates a further complication. In 1983, the Department of Health and Social Security (DHSS) established 28 care management demonstration projects to help long-stay hospital patients (e.g. the mentally ill, those with learning disabilities) move to community settings. Cambridge (1992) has documented the diversity of approaches adopted by these projects and devised a seven category typology which shows that one important axis of differentiation was the location of the care management (e.g. social services, health care or multidisciplinary care).

This illustrates the complexity of meaning which can underlie a very simple and apparently technical and unambiguous term such as 'care management'. There is considerable uncertainty as to how local authorities should precede. The enormity of the task has been recognized and is summarized in a report by the Audit Commission (1992). Several commentators have highlighted the slow progress that is being made (Allen, Daley and Leat, 1992; Hoyes and Means, 1993). This progress will continue to be slow until local authorities tackle the questions about which style of care management they wish to implement and the subsequent questions such as who does it, do they hold the budget and should assessment be separate from the management of the care package.

COMMISSIONING

Commissioning of services, the contracting and purchasing of social care services, is a very new role for local authorities who, prior to the NHSCCA Act had largely been direct providers of care services. Local authorities are therefore experiencing a very marked change in their role from providers of care to enabling authorities. In this capacity they have a number of roles to fulfil. The Department of Health Guide on purchasing and contracting describes these as 'to identify the needs for care among the population it serves, plan how best to meet those needs, set overall strategies, priorities and targets, commission and purchase as well as provide necessary services and ensure their quality and value.' (DoH/SSI, 1991c, para. 4.3).

It is through the commissioning role that central government ensures that local authorities will create and stimulate the 'mixed' economy of care which is then regulated by the contracting and quality assurance mechanisms. Local authorities were obliged in the three years up to and including 1995/96 to spend 85% of the special transition grant (the money transferred from the social security budget to local authorities, which is discussed later in this chapter) in the private/voluntary sector, purchasing and commissioning services which will then be used in the care packages put together for individual clients. The rationale behind the creation of the welfare market and the increased use of private/voluntary providers is to encourage competition between providers in the hope that this will result in increased value for money and better quality services.

In order to implement the purchasing and contracting requirements local authorities have, as noted earlier, had to reorganize their internal structures to reflect these different activities. As the Department of Health (1989, p. 23) noted, to make contracting work would 'require a clear distinction to be made between the purchasing and providing functions within a local authority'. Where local authorities continue to be direct care providers of, for example, home care or residential care, these functions are now separate from the purchasing arm of the authority. Indeed, some authorities have transferred their direct service provision to specially created organizations. This split in function would ensure equality of treatment for different providers and serve to 'distance' care managers from directly provided services so that they did not feel obliged to use them. This parallels the changes which have taken place within the health sector.

It is again fairly easy to state that local authorities should separate out provider and purchaser functions, but how is this to be achieved in practical terms? As with care management there is no single universally accepted model of the local authority purchaser/provider spilt for the provision of community care.

Price Waterhouse (1991) conducted a review for the Department of Health which identified three potential approaches to the implementation of the purchaser/provider division. These were distinguished by the 'level' within the organization at which the separation occurred; at strategic level, senior management level (where the director held the only combined post) and at local (area team) level. Each model has its advantages and disadvantages. In the first model there is minimal disruption to the working of the organization, but no clear separation of functions envisaged by the changes. Model two involves clear separation of functions but is very centralized. Model three is the most responsive to local needs but is the most organizationally complex and may involve considerable duplication of effort within any authority. Means and Smith (1995) note that progress towards the implementation of the purchaser/provider split has been slow and with authorities preferring to see purchasing as a central function rather than one which was devolved to local level. Of course this pattern of service organization may well change as the experience of the implementation of the community care changes increases.

Contracting

The period after 1991 has seen the development of the new field of health and social care contracting. There are three main types of contracts:

- Block contracts involve an agency in purchasing a certain amount of service for a given price. This gives a guaranteed income to the provider but may result in purchases paying for services not used and limit the choice of individuals.
- Spot contracts involve the purchase of individual services as when they are required.
- Cost and volume contracts are half way between the two; the authority buys a minimum amount of service with the ability to purchase additional units if required.

Regardless of the type of contract each will contain quite lengthy specifications setting out what is expected of the provider. Monitoring these specifications is one way of ensuring the quality of the services provided.

The implementation of the contracting culture has fundamentally altered the nature of the relationship between local authorities and the voluntary sector. In the past, local authorities gave grants to voluntary agencies. However these grants were not usually tied to delivery of specific services, such as the provision of meals or places at a day-centre, but were usually a general way of recognizing the contribution of the voluntary group. There are worries that by being 'forced' into the role of contracted service providers the ability of the voluntary sector to act as independent advocates or to innovate with new ways of providing and organizing care will be reduced. Furthermore contract specifications may require providers to use staff with specified minimum levels of training; this could be problematic for a voluntary agency which relied upon volunteers to provide services. Hence, the introduction of the social care market, the contracting system as well as the changed nature of local authorities will also alter the way that voluntary sector organizations function and are managed.

It is the stated intention of the community care changes to develop a 'mixed economy' of care by stimulating the private sector. Private operators are, as we have already noted, major players in the nursing home/residential home sectors. However the domiciliary sector is less well developed. Overall, the distribution of private sector care in the UK is very uneven. Some areas, such as the south coast, have significant clusters of private care homes while in many inner city districts there are few such enterprises. Also, many private sector providers are small businesses. For them, like many voluntary agencies, the staff and resource requirements needed to become involved in the contracting culture may be too onerous.

How successful has the development of the mixed economy of care been? It is of course very early on in the implementation of the community care changes to be definitive about this. Progress towards this objective is slow partly because the size of the private/voluntary sector in each local authority varies so markedly. Has the development of the market achieved its stated aims of improving consumer choice? Meredith (1995) is of the opinion that due to financial considerations there has been little extra benefit to consumers in the form of increased choice about services received. She notes that the exception to this is for those users who are able and willing to use their own financial resources to augment the contribution from the public sector.

QUALITY ASSURANCE

Quality assurance relates to the obligation of local authorities to ensure the quality of the services they provide/purchase. Three separate strands are brought together under this heading; complaints procedures, inspection and contract monitoring.

Complaints procedures

As we have already seen, much of the rhetoric of the community care changes has been towards increasing the voice of users and carers. Complaints are one way of gauging how well services are doing and can provide a crude quality assurance mechanism. Under the NHSCCA, local authorities are required to establish and publish procedures by which users and carers can register their complaints. A report of complaints received must be presented annually to the social services committee. However the existence of a publicized procedure does not guarantee the user/carer redress. Meredith (1995) provides a very comprehensive review of the structure and working of the complaints system.

Inspection units are 'arms length' units which were initially charged with the responsibility for 'inspecting and reporting on both local authority and registered independent residential care homes' (DoH, 1989, p. 45). Prior to the NHSCCA, local authorities had had a duty to register and inspect independent homes but *not* those for which they had direct responsibility (i.e. those provided under part three of the 1948 National Assistance Act). This led to the charge that local authorities set standards for private and voluntary homes which were not achieved in their own establishments. Health authorities remain responsible for the registration and inspection of nursing homes. Dually registered homes are registered and inspected by both agencies.

What do inspection units do and how do they achieve the tasks set for them? Like almost every other facet of community care, there is enormous variation between authorities in how these units function. Inspection units work with residential homes is largely based upon the duties laid down in the 1984 Registered Homes Act. The main tasks are as follows;

- registration of residential homes;
- inspection of homes with four or more residents;
- improving the quality of care;
- setting standards which homes are expected to meet;

- make publicly available reports about individual inspections and the work of the unit;
- develop a policy for following up inspections;
- seeking the views of users and cares;
- feeding back the results of inspections to the purchasing/contracting process.

Meredith (1995) provides a very detailed and comprehensive review of the registration and inspection process.

There is very little provision for the inspection of day-care services or services provided in people's homes. Indeed, there is no statutory requirement for these types of services to be inspected although the people receiving such services may be every bit as vulnerable and frail as those in residential/nursing home care. There is some limited scope for the maintenance of minimum standards through the complaints and contract monitoring mechanisms. However it would seem desirable to develop some requirement for domiciliary services to be brought within the registration and inspection procedures.

The final strand of the quality assurance web is through contract monitoring. Contract specification and monitoring are very time consuming and labour intensive activities. Furthermore although local authorities are required to monitor the quality of services as part of the contracting process this is actually extremely difficult to achieve. How is quality, especially in a very complex area such as the provision of social care, to be specified in a form which is relatively easy to monitor. It is fairly straightforward to set some criteria such as numbers of staff, qualifications of staff employed or hours of care. This area remains one of the biggest challenges faced by local authorities in implementing the NHSCCA.

COMMUNITY CARE: FUNDING ARRANGEMENTS

Before moving on to consider some of the substantive areas concerning the provision of community care for older people it is necessary to review, very briefly, the area of financial arrangements for community care. We will concentrate upon three specific aspects of the arrangements; the general allocation of funds to local authorities, the special transition grant and the arrangements for long-term care.

General funding for local authorities

In Britain, local authorities raise a certain amount of money through the council tax system. However, this is insufficient to cover all their financial commitments. Money for local authorities is allocated by central government from the general taxation budget to help them pay for the services that they provide. The last two decades have been ones of financial stringency in which central government has sought to contain both national and local government expenditure. This has meant that the implementation of the community care changes has taken place at a time of considerable financial restrictions.

Each local authority receives a block grant from central government. The amount of money which is to be made available to local government is not based upon any 'objective' assessment of the need for resources by local authorities. Rather it is the result of a political decision made by ministers and the treasury about how much they can afford to spend. The block grant contains assumptions made by the Department of the Environment about how much local authorities should be spending on their main services, such as social services. These are termed standard spending assessments (SSAs). Each SSA specifies what the Department of the Environment determines as the amount of money that an authority should spend (e.g. on social services).

Standard spending assessments

Standard spending assessments (SSAs) for social services were first introduced in 1990/1991. Again these are not based upon local needs but are a mechanism for distributing money from central to local government. The social services SSA is divided into three blocks; children under 18 years of age (35.5% of the total), elderly people (45.2%) and other adults who need support (19.3%). How are these SSAs reached? Each component of the social services SSA is calculated by a formulae which relates to population and demographic factors and 'deprivation' index (such as the number of pensioners living alone) calculated from the 1991 census data. However, the relevance of the deprivation factors used as an indicator of the 'need' for social services expenditure is open to debate.

Means and Smith (1995) suggest that the system is open to two major criticisms. First, they suggest that the overall sums allocated from central government are totally inadequate to meet the stated objectives of the community care changes. They argue that this has resulted in the implementation of the reforms at a time of financial stringency. Second, they argue that the system is flawed because of the variations in allocations between authorities, with apparently similar circumstances, which the distribution system reveals.

These assessments are, however, not mandatory. They simply represent the amount of money central government thinks (or suggests) a local authority should spend. The allocation of money between services (e.g. social services, education and housing) is a decision which is made at local level. Hence funds for community care are not ring-fenced and are subject to the influence of local political decision-making. Hence in a climate of financial stringency authorities are faced with stark choices; reduce the level of services so that they are provided for an increasingly tightly defined client group or attempt to increase revenue by increased charging for services.

The special transition grant (STG)

The engine driving the community care changes was the vast unplanned expenditure from the social security budget on private residential and nursing home care.

One objective of the reforms was to transfer money from the social security budget to the local authorities. This transfer of money has been the subject of considerable debate both about the amount transferred and how it is then allocated between authorities. These debates mirror those described above with regard to the SSA for social services and again it is uncertain as to how these financial decisions will effect older people and the types of services they receive.

Charging for community care services

To conclude our brief review of the financial basis of community care we must now consider how these changes affect older people. There have always been a minority of older people who have paid for the services they receive, either at home or in residential/nursing homes. Those who do receive care which is funded entirely out of their own resources are largely unaffected by these changes.

We will not consider here the position of those in long-stay care before the imposition of the community care changes as this unnecessarily complicates the situation. Here we will confine our attention to describing the position for those who wished to enter care after April 1st 1993. Those who wish to enter residential or nursing home care but who cannot afford to pay for it have to undergo an assessment of their need for such care. If the need for such care is accepted then the local authority will place the person in care. A means test is then undertaken to establish how much the person must contribute towards their care. A similar system operates for entry into nursing home care, except where the NHS accepts responsibility for long-term care provision when it is free.

This highlights a recurrent theme that, for those who need nursing care, there is a distinction between those who are accepted as the responsibility of the NHS (when the care is provided free) and those who are not (when the older persons must contribute towards their care). There are many rules and regulations concerning how people are assessed and it is not necessary to go into detail as these are covered elsewhere (Meredith, 1995). However some points are important to note. First, under certain circumstances the value of an older person's house is included in their assessment of their financial assets. This has caused concern because of the desire of many older people 'to leave something for their children'. It is also being seen as a 'penalty' for being thrifty in their younger years. Clearly this is at odds with the stated desire of the government to see 'wealth trickle down between the generations'. Second, when financial circumstances are assessed for domiciliary services the value of the house is not taken into account. Here is the beginning of another perverse incentive whereby very frail elderly people will wish to be maintained at home (when it is clearly unsatisfactory to do so) because they do not wish to loose their home by entering care. The implementation of these new funding rules has resulted in the stimulation of debate about how long-term care should be funded and we will return to this issue (Chapter 7).

As we have seen above, there has always been an acceptance of the position of 'charging' residents for local authority residential home care. Those entering such homes have always undergone a strict means test to assess their ability to contribute towards their care. Charging for domiciliary care services has always been less accepted and less widespread. However this is now emerging as a key element to the implementation of the community care reforms as it represents one way of generating income.

The 1991 act did not radically alter the position for local authorities with respect to paying for non-residential services. Local authorities are allowed to set their own charges for services but these must be 'reasonable'. Means and Smith (1995) identify three positions adopted by local authorities with respect to charging for domiciliary services. These are:

- to preserve the principle of free services;
- to increase charges in relation to the income of the recipient (but not necessarily to the level of service received);
- to cost the level of services provided and then relate this to the financial status of the recipient.

Again, each authority is free to respond to perceived financial pressures as they wish but it seems inevitable that the issue of charging for domiciliary services will become more common and that users will be required to bear the 'true' cost of services rather than a nominal amount. This of course implies that older people have the ability to pay for such care. This is an issue we will return to (Chapter 3).

CONCLUSION

In this chapter we have provided an overview of the implementation of community care and described the main changes resulting from the implementation of the NHSCCA. It is, of course, far too soon after the implementation of these changes to issue a definitive statement upon the success (or otherwise) of the implementation. As we have seen, local authorities have had to implement these changes in a time of considerable financial uncertainty. Furthermore implementation has been hampered by political uncertainty, uncertainty about the structure of local government because of an ongoing review about the structure of local government and because of substantial changes in other areas of local governments workload such as the implementation of the 1989 Children Act. In the following chapters we will examine in more detail some of the issues raised.

Assessing the need for community care at a population level

3

INTRODUCTION

As we have already seen, resources for community care (as well as health services) are constrained and indeed the new policy has been implemented in a time of financial stringency. In the health field there is a lively debate about how the resources available for health care should be spent. This is complemented by an increased awareness of the need to describe, or profile, the characteristics of the populations served by these different agencies and to try to assess the health care needs of particular populations (Stevens and Raferty, 1994, Pickin and St Leger, 1993). The trend towards the development of health needs assessment and population profiling is related to the move towards explicit rationing and prioritization of health service provision. It is also related to the examination of the most appropriate mix of skills, both between and within professional groups, required to provide these services.

Within the community care setting assessment of need is to be conducted at both the individual and community level. As has been stated in the White Paper (DoH, 1989), local authorities are expected to 'assess the needs of the population they serve'. Population level needs assessment is seen as being an essential prerequisite to effective service planning. However guidance on this was issued in late 1993 some time after the implementation of the changes (DoH, 1993). In this chapter we will be reviewing macro level community care needs assessment and reviewing the main factors which are important in determining current (and future needs) for community care. Needs assessment at the micro (or individual level) will be discussed in Chapter 4.

COMMUNITY CARE PLANS AND POPULATION NEEDS ASSESSMENT

The community care reforms require each local authority to draw up a community care plan annually. These plans are required to state explicit objectives and priorities for community care and set targets for achieving these. Such plans are public documents and as such are available for scrutiny by members of the general public. Central government issues guidance on how local authorities should undertake the preparation of their community care and this guidance has changed over time to reflect increased experience of community care.

The first clutch of community care plans in 1992 should have covered the following areas:

- an assessment of the needs of the local population and the specific client groups for whom they intended to provide services;
- details of current services and plans for development;
- identification of priorities;
- quality assurance;
- development of consumer choice;
- methods of stimulating the mixed economy resources (both staffing and costs);
- details of consultation;
- plans for dissemination.

Further guidance on the contents of community care plans have been given in the 'Foster-Laming' and the 'Laming-Langlands' letters (DoH, 1992). These letters laid out a series of key tasks which local authorities were expected to achieve. The Foster-Laming letter of 1992 specifically charged that the 1993 community care plans should cover the following issues:

- resources available;
- services available;
- assessment procedures (including financial circumstances);
- arrangements for the purchase of residential and nursing home care;
- charging policies;
- details of arrangements with other agencies involved in community care (including GP fundholders);
- consumer choice and arrangements for dissemination.

The joint letters from the Social Services Inspectorate and NHS Executive (the Laming-Langlands letters) in May 1993 stressed the key tasks of:

- increasing user and care involvement;
- developing assessment and care management;
- developing joint work with health authorities;
- developing relationships with providers;
- developing non-residential services;

- involving housing agencies in community care.

A central and consistent element of the community care plans has focused upon the assessment of need at the population level and this issue is now considered in more detail.

What is needs assessment?

Before considering the social care context, it is necessary to review briefly the development of health needs assessment, as much of the work in this area has taken place within a health context. We also need to define the terms which are used when considering the areas of needs assessment. Like the term community care, needs assessment is also a term which can have a variety of different meanings.

In recent years there has been a significant move towards the development of ways of assessing the health care needs of populations. The Department of Health recognized in 1988 that 'the provision of health services should be informed by an assessment of health needs' (Pickin and St Leger, 1993). However the strongest stimulus for a move towards health needs assessment was the 1989 reform of the NHS, and the introduction of the purchaser/provider split.

In order to purchase appropriate health care for its resident population, health commissioning agencies need to profile, or describe, the characteristics of its population and assess its need for health care and then purchase appropriate health care. Such tasks are the responsibility of the public health departments. The results of these activities are often made available in the reports of the Director of Public Health and the purchasing plans and intentions of the agencies. Similarly, the community care reforms have stimulated the development of population (and individual) level assessment of social care needs. Indeed, there is a link between these two levels of assessment as individual assessments may form the building blocks for the development of population profiles.

Needs assessment: defining the key terms

Before we can explore the issue of needs assessment we must first clarify the terms that are being used in the discussion. As McWalter *et al.* (1994) note, it is essential to have clear definitions of the terms so that suitable tools may be developed to collect the relevant information. Within a health service context it is usual, considering the very broad areas of needs assessment and client group profiling, to distinguish between three very important concepts; need, demand and supply. Such a distinction is also useful within the social care context.

The terms need, demand and supply are often used interchangeably in popular discourse, but they have a very specific meaning when discussing population level assessments of needs. Within this context the terms may be defined as follows:

- *need* defines interventions/treatments or services from which people (either individuals or populations) would gain benefit;

- *demand* relates to what people would use in a free, social care system (or pay for in a market based system);
- *supply* describes what is actually provided.

Each of these three terms is now considered in more detail.

Need

Need is a word which is very commonly used in everyday conversation. The Shorter Oxford Dictionary defines need as 'to be in want of'. Within a population health context need has a more specific and technical meaning: the ability of an individual (or population) to benefit from a specific health care intervention (Stevens and Raferty 1994). Within the health care context such benefits are termed 'outcomes'. These are used to measure the success (or otherwise) of an intervention in achieving its stated goals. For example, how well does an early discharge scheme meet its desired objective of reducing length of stay. This, of course, requires that services have very clearly stated goals which they wish to achieve (we will return to this issue in the very brief consideration of evaluation later in this chapter). An outcome describes the result of an intervention and within the health care field there has been an explosion of interest in the development and use of outcome measures (Jinkinson, 1994). Similarly, the need for social care is defined as the ability of an individual or population to benefit from care and is contingent upon the existence of effective services, therapies or interventions to remedy the identified problem. As yet, however, there has been less development in the field of social care outcome measures, although some of the health based measures are applicable within a social care setting.

If need is defined in terms of what people would benefit from, this raises the question of how we define benefit (or outcome). There is no consensus as to how benefit should be measured, although its multifaceted nature is widely accepted in both the health and social care fields. Within the health field it is usual to measure benefit (or outcome) in a variety of domains including mortality (i.e. survival), morbidity (i.e. symptoms) and quality of life. In the areas of morbidity measurement and quality of life measurement, there have been considerable interest in the development of standardized outcome measures which can be used in a variety of different settings and with different population groups (e.g. older people). Within a social care context it has been suggested that there are two important aspects which should be included in any definition of the benefits from social care interventions. These are: (restoration/maximization of) independence; and quality of life (McWalter *et al.*, 1994).

In the social care field, it is important that the term 'benefit' is interpreted widely to include the perspective of both users and carers. This makes the evaluation of social care interventions more complex (see below). However, to exclude the perspective of carers would give us only a very partial perspective on the outcomes resultant from services.

It is also important to remember that 'need' is a dynamic concept. Services which were 'needed' in the past, such as mass chest X–ray screening or the provision of mobile meals services to people whose houses had been bombed during the war may outlive their usefulness. The development of new and worthwhile services and interventions will create new social care needs.

In the health field, this very broad concept of need is usually further subdivided into four components (Bradshaw,1972). The basis of the classification is how the health care needs are distinguished and this typology may be usefully applied to the field of social care at both individual and population levels of assessment. Bradshaw (1972) distinguishes between different sorts of need:

- *Normative needs* are those defined or identified by an expert or professional. This involves them in defining a 'standard' below which people are described as being 'in need'. For example, a home help organizer who considers that an older person needs help with house care is a normative based needs assessment.
- *Felt needs* are those needs that are identified by users or carers. These are needs identified by users such as requiring help with gardening or house maintenance. This aspect of need would be central to any individual needs assessment.
- *Expressed needs* are felt needs translated into action, for example the demand from older people for a 'drop-in' centre or from minority elders for special dietary provisions.
- *Comparative needs* are defined by the comparison of social care provision received by the population (or subsection of the population) in one area, with those elsewhere. If we do not know what the optimal pattern of service provision is then simple comparisons between groups and areas may highlight areas of unmet (or over met) need. The comparative approach is especially powerful in the context of population level community care needs assessment. For example, studies of comparative need may highlight differences between areas in access to domiciliary or residential care provision.

Demand

Demand for social health care relates to needs translated into action. It is what is asked for. Demand may originate from users, carers, voluntary workers or professionals (or indeed some combination of these).

The demand for social care services is not necessarily an accurate reflection of the need for services because demands for services are affected by the following:

- knowledge of the existence of services. This very simply reflects the fact that an individual cannot use or demand a service if they are unaware of its existence. For example, older people cannot attend a 'drop-in' lunch club if they don't know it exists. Inevitably, publicity, whether at local or national level, about the existence of a service will increase demands for that service;
- the local availability of services. This means that if a service does not exist locally or is limited in its availability then demand is affected. For example a respite care service which only operates in a very restricted manner is not likely to attract great use.

Supply

Supply relates to the availability of particular services, but again is not a surrogate for the need of social care. The level of supply of a particular service reflects numerous pressures and constraints including historical patterns of supply, as well as political, professional and public pressure.

The fact that some services are available may well stimulate use even though they may not be appropriate for meeting peoples needs. The importance of supply side factors in generating utilization of some services should not be under-estimated, although its exact impact remains difficult to quantify, and probably varies between different services. However, one of the main features of the community care changes is to get away from a 'supply' based identification and meeting of individuals needs.

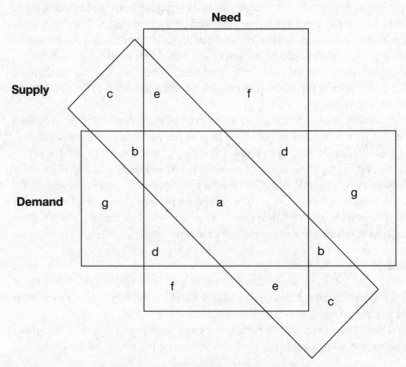

Figure 3.1 The relationship between need, demand and supply (after Stevens and Raferty, 1994)

The relationship between need, demand and supply

What is the relationship between need, demand and supply? It has already been hinted that the relationship between demand, supply and need is not symmetrical. There are seven main combinations of the concepts of need, demand and supply (Figure 3.1).

The different combinations are outlined below:

- intervention or services needed, wanted and supplied;
- some services will be demanded and supplied but are not needed;
- some services may be provided but are not needed or demanded;
- some services will be needed and demanded but not supplied;
- services needed and supplied but not demanded;
- services which are needed but not demanded or supplied (known as unmet need – see below);
- services may be demanded by individuals or groups but are neither needed or supplied.

Services that are needed but not demanded or supplies may be divided broadly into three main groups.

Unmet needs

Unmet needs are those where there is a need but no demand or supply. There may be extensive needs existing within the community which are neither identified by social care workers nor services provided for them. This is well illustrated by surveys of elderly people living in the community which inevitably and universally identify extensive amounts of previously unrecorded illness, morbidity or need for services (Williamson *et al.*, 1964).

Overmet needs

'Overmet' needs are those where there is supply but either no demand or need. However, identifying such services can be problematic as there is often considerable professional investment in them and to reduce them is often very contentious involving as it does 'a cut' in provision.

Demand without need or supply

These services again highlight the contentious nature of needs assessment work. Because, as well as identifying areas where there is unmet need for services, unnecessary/inappropriate forms of provision may be identified. Questioning the *status quo* of service provision can be a challenging and uncomfortable experience.

EVALUATION OF SOCIAL CARE

The whole basis of needs assessment is the provision of services/therapies/interventions which are of proven benefit to the users/clients/patients. This then raises the problem of what interventions are beneficial and how this is determined. Although there is much more interest now being expressed in the importance of evaluation in health care (St Leger *et al.*, 1992), it remains unfortunate that remarkably few health services have been evaluated. It has been estimated that only 20% of health service interventions have been evaluated and found to be of proven benefit (St Leger *et al.*, 1992). In the field of community care/social care it is likely that even fewer interventions have been evaluated. This section raises some issues and questions about evaluation which are pertinent to the development of community care based needs assessment and profiling, but it is obviously only the most sketchy introduction to this vast and complex area of research.

The first thing we need to determine is what is evaluation? In this context, evaluation relates to the 'scientific' assessment of the extent to which community care services (or their constituent parts) achieve their stated goals. Thus, a prerequisite of any evaluation is that the service/intervention under review should have clearly stated and measurable goals. For example, do domiciliary services prevent admission to long-stay care or do respite care schemes reduce the burden felt by carers?

In attempting to evaluate any health care intervention Maxwell (1984) suggests that six issues need to be addressed. These six issues are pertinent to the study of social and community care interventions, and are discussed below.

Effectiveness
This is the 'key' aspect of any evaluation in that it describes the achievement in terms of specified outcomes resulting from the intervention. This measure tells us how successful (or otherwise) an intervention was in achieving its stated goals. For example, the number of older people 'prevented' from admission to long-stay care by the development of an intensive home care service. This, of course, requires that all services/interventions have clearly articulated and measurable goals. This is not always the case.

Efficiency
This is an economically based measure and describes the relationship between the resources put in, and the outputs from a service. This is a very difficult concept to measure in social care based studies. However, it is worth noting that services can be both efficient but also ineffective.

Equity
This examines the degree to which the service/intervention is offered equally to all those who need it. For example, a home meals service, by only providing a limited range of foods, may exclude users from various cultural backgrounds.

Acceptability
This is a neglected but important concept in both needs assessment work and evaluation studies, but it is one which should be at the forefront. If the social care system is unacceptable to potential users, then regardless of its effectiveness or level of efficiency it will not be used. This dimension of evaluation deals with the way in which a treatment or service is delivered and is largely concerned with issues of quality. Is it delivered humanely? What do users think of the service? Would you be happy for one of your family to be cared for in this way? Issues such

as providing culturally appropriate care fall within the broad concept of acceptability. This is a difficult but vital aspect of evaluation to measure.

Appropriateness

This relates to the selection of the 'most appropriate' method of treatment or service delivery for a particular health care problem or client group. An intervention can only be appropriate when certain criteria are met. The intervention should only be performed if appropriate and adequate resources are available, and in a way which is acceptable to the patient. For example getting young offenders to undertake house maintenance for older people could be an inappropriate way of delivering a 'care and repair' type service if the older people were not happy with the system or the service providers lacked the necessary skills.

Accessibility

This relates to the access of services and considers whether individuals get the treatment that they need. Again this is a multifaceted concept as it relates to the barriers which may (or may not) exist for people using services, such as distance to services, transport, access for disabled people and the operation and opening hours of offices. Other aspects of the concept of accessibility include access to the decision making process and access to information about community care matters in general and the services offered. For the various aspects of access there are issues regarding the right of access, the ease of access and the cost of access, which require consideration.

When looking at community care intervention with older people we need to consider how far each of these issues are addressed. It is clearly difficult to define indicators to measure all of these aspects but a comprehensive evaluation study should try to assess these dimensions. When reviewing evaluative studies critically, we also need to look at how these different areas have been assessed.

WHAT SHOULD BE INCLUDED IN A POPULATION LEVEL NEEDS ASSESSMENT?

According to the Department of Health Policy guidance, community care plans should 'identify the care needs of the local population taking into account factors which are age distribution, problems associated with living in inner city areas or rural areas, special needs of ethnic minority communities, the number of homeless and transient people likely to require care'. In this section we will consider some of the methodological issues involved in population level needs assessment and the sources of data available.

Need is defined as the ability of an individual or collection of individuals to benefit from care. This is problematic in the social care field because so few interventions, such as home helps, home meals services or day care, have been rigorously evaluated. However, any comprehensive needs assessment should include a review of effective service interventions. Such reviews are now becoming an important element of health care purchasing especially with the growing trend towards 'evidence based medicine'. Critical appraisal skills and the critical review of the nature of service interventions through the development of systematic reviews are likely to become increasingly important within the social care field.

In the context of community care, population based needs assessment is concerned with estimating, projecting and classifying the needs of a local population. One way of identifying needs is to try to establish the number of people in a population who may be experiencing difficulties with maintaining an independent life in the community. Several sources of data including demographic information, national surveys and local surveys may be used to provide information about the need for community care by populations. Some of these sources of data may provide direct evidence about the distribution of specific problems which directly relate to the need for care services (e.g. the number of people who are unable to undertake self-care activities (such as feeding, washing and dressing). Other sources of data provide indirect (or proxy) measures of need such as the percentage of very old people (i.e. aged 85 years and over) living alone. It is assumed these people are more likely to experience disability and are less likely to have access to informal carers or have a reduced network of informal carers. Clearly, working within this framework, the needs are identified regardless of whether these needs are ever presented to the appropriate authorities.

Methodological aspects of population based needs assessment

Incidence and prevalence

In population based needs assessment, two very important concepts, originally derived from epidemiological studies, are those of incidence and prevalence. The method of calculation of these two measures is shown in Table 3.1.

Table 3.1 Method of calculation of incidence and prevalence rates

$$\text{a) Incidence} = \frac{\text{the number of new cases in a given reference period}}{\text{population at risk}}$$

e.g. Calculation of incidence rate for dementia in those aged 65 years and over

$$= \frac{\text{number of new cases in one year/population aged 65 years and over}}{200/20000 = 1\% \text{ (or 10 per 1000)}}$$

$$\text{b) Prevalence} = \frac{\text{total number of people aged 65 years and over with dementia}}{\text{population at risk}}$$

e.g. Calculation of dementia prevalence rate

$$= \frac{\text{total numbers with dementia/population aged 65 years and over}}{500/20000 = 2.5\% \text{ (or 25 per 1000)}}$$

Incidence describes the number of new cases of a specific disease (or disability) occurring within a defined population (e.g. a local authority area) during a given time period (e.g. a year). Although typically used to describe the number of new cases of a disease, it is easy to see that the notion of incidence has a wider applicability, as it could also be used to describe the number of newly disabled people each year or the number of children entering/leaving care. Clearly, in undertaking needs assessment we need to have some indication of the number of people who might be referred for assessment. Put another way, the incidence rate describes the number of new cases that a social care agency might expect over a given period. This can be used to estimate the 'expected' workload of a department and the potential requirement for funds. Hence it is important to be able to estimate incidence rates.

Prevalence records the number of cases of a specific disease (e.g. stroke) in a defined population at a specific time. The prevalence of a specific condition illustrates the total workload which a social services department may be dealing with at any single point.

Although incidence and prevalence rates are usually used to measure disease, it is easy to see that they may also be used to describe issues relevant to the development of population based community care needs assessment. For example, we may calculate the number of new disabled elderly people (incidence rate) as well as the prevalence of disability in particular areas or populations. This would indicate both the number of new cases we might have to deal with each year, as well as enumerating the total workload for this client group.

Incidence rates are extremely useful measures for those concerned with needs assessment, as they indicate how many new cases of a disability, or particular form of behaviour (such as hospital admission) might be expected over a particular time period. Changes in incidence rates indicate whether a particular problem is increasing (or decreasing) and also reflect the changing size of the 'population at risk' of particular social care problems. Incidence rates could form a useful measure for the evaluation of the effectiveness of many social care based activities. It may be inferred that decreasing incidence rates indicate the success of particular interventions. For example, a reduced incidence of admissions to nursing home care may be ascribed to the development of intensive home care services.

However, it is worth noting that both the notions of incidence and prevalence are problematic, because they assume that we may unambiguously categorize populations (or individuals) into two distinct and discrete groups – those with the disability and those without. For many conditions especially those which are of interest to those involved in the need for community care, this is difficult because there are rarely situations in which individuals may be unambiguously described as having or lacking the condition under review. This is particularly problematic for chronic conditions such as dementia or disability where there is a continuum ranging from no impairment to total impairment.

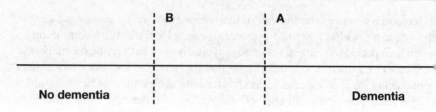

Figure 3.2 The case definition threshold

Deciding at which point along the continuum (Figure 3.2) dementia or disability are defined (known as the case definition threshold) will greatly influence the size of the identified problem and hence the incidence/prevalence rates. There will be far fewer disabled within the population if the threshold is at point B instead of point A.

Applying national data to local populations

It will be seen later in this chapter that there are a variety of data sources which are available for local authority areas and which may be used to build up a profile of the social care needs of specific populations, such as older people or young mothers.

However, some data are only available nationally (or for nationally representative sample populations). However, these data may also be applied to local populations in order to estimate the extent of a particular problem such as disabling stroke or dementia. For example, Table 3.2 illustrates how data about the prevalence of dementia among older people have been used to estimate the number of people (or prevalence) of this disease in a hypothetical social services locality. Using a similar methodology it would be possible to estimate the number of newly disabled or demented elderly people (i.e. the incidence) occurring in a specific population.

Table 3.2 Estimated number of people aged 60 years and over with dementia: Great Britain 1996–2021

Age	% with dementia	population (000s) 1996	2021	estimated cases 1996	2021	% increase 1996–2021[a]
60–64	0.5	2699	3844	13 495	19 220	42
65–69	1.1	2578	3219	28 358	35 409	25
70–74	3.9	2356	3171	91 884	123 669	36
75–79	6.7	1782	2272	119 394	152 224	27
80–84	13.5	1282	1497	173 070	202 095	18
85–89	22.8	727	919	165 756	209 532	26
90+	34.1	340	672	115 940	229 152	98
All 60+	–	11 764	15 594	707 897	971 301	32

[a]Dementia prevalence rates derived from: Jorm, *et al*.., 1987

COMMUNITY CASE NEEDS ASSESSMENT: SOURCES OF DATA

The starting point for any needs assessment is the development of a population profile which will describe the basic features of the local population (DoH, 1993). This exercise should be undertaken for all the potential client groups for community care (e.g. those with learning disabilities or HIV) but our examples will be concerned with only older people (although the principles apply across the spectrum). Three basic sets of data will be required for a comprehensive population based needs assessment: population data, population projections and data about the prevalence and incidence of conditions that are likely to influence an elderly person's ability to live independently in the community. In this section we will consider the availability of the main sources of data and their limitations.

Demographic data

The most basic information required for any form of 'needs assessment' is the size and composition of the population under review. Accurate population data are fundamental to the development of sound needs assessment as these both indicate the size of particular client groups that are of interest (e.g. older people). They provide the denominators for the calculation of both incidence and prevalence rates described earlier. The population census is the source of our most accurate and detailed population data.

In England and Wales, since the first complete census in 1801, there has been a full census every 10 years (with the exception of 1941). The last population census took place in 1991. The aim of the census is to provide a full count of the population and to collect data about the main characteristics of the population, such as age and sex structure. The census is conducted, analysed and disseminated by a government department, the Office of National Statistics (ONS) (formerly the Office of Population Censuses and Surveys (OPCS)).

The precise data collected varies from census to census, but always includes basic demographic information, such as age, sex, marital condition, place of birth, occupation, number of children, usual place of residence and length of present residence. The 1991 census included two new pieces of information, never previously collected, namely self-defined ethnic origin and a question about chronic health problems. Data are also collected about details of the residence (including its type, tenure, accommodation and facilities), employment, migration and care ownership. The census does not collect data about the financial circumstances of the population

Although it is a legal requirement that people should complete census forms, the census does not manage to enumerate everybody. It is estimated that, in 1991, 2% of the population were not included in the census. This is important because this percentage is not equally distributed across the population. That is, certain groups are more likely than others to have not been enumerated, thereby introducing bias (or non-representativeness) into the resultant statistical data. Specific groups or geographical areas are systematically under-represented by the census. Minority groups, those living in the inner city, men aged 16–29 years of age and those aged 85 and over had the highest rates of census non-completion in 1991. Nationally, it has been estimated that one million people were missed by the census.

As the census only takes place every decade, then information that is routinely used in undertaking needs assessment work can become out-of-date. While there are estimates of the way the size and age–sex composition of the population is changing between censuses, there are no ways of routinely reviewing the accuracy of data about the social characteristics of the population. For instance, revised estimates of the size and demographic composition of, for example, minority communities, are not made available.

For planning purposes, it is often essential to have some idea of the likely size and composition of the population in years to come. The essential difference between population estimates and population projections is that an *estimate* is based on knowledge of the births, deaths and migration that have happened, and a *projection* is based upon what is thought likely to happen. Therefore assumptions are made about trends in mortality, birth rates and migration. These projections are likely to be less reliable the further into the future they are made, because the assumptions about birth and death rates are likely to become increasingly inaccurate. When researching the future age composition of populations there are important limitations. For example, we can estimate the number of elderly people in 2020 based upon our data about existing patterns of mortality. Projecting what percentage of the population this will represent is more problematic as this entails making assumptions about future patterns of fertility which are always very unreliable.

Sources of information about health and disability

Information about the incidence and prevalence of conditions which may effect an older person's ability to live independently in the community may be derived from a variety of sources. These may be broadly divided into two types:

- national data sets;
- locally based information, such as health or disability surveys.

Most of the examples described in this section relate to national data. However this does not mean that local data sets are unimportant although their availability and quality does vary considerably. When using local surveys as a way of estimating the prevalence of specific conditions such as disability users need to evaluate critically the quality of data. This is done by examining sampling (i.e. were responders drawn from the general population or was the survey based upon samples of service users), response rate (are the data limited by non-response), bias (the systematic under-representation of specific groups) and the types of questions used (were leading questions used or were standardized assessment schedules modified thereby undermining their scientific properties).

Information about disability and disabling conditions

When attempting to assess the needs of older people for community care we are interested in data that relate to the difficulties experienced by people in maintaining their independence. Hence we are predominantly interested in establishing the prevalence (and incidence) of disability, and disabling conditions (both mental and physical) in population rather than in describing health status *per se*. What sources of data are available for use in community care population profiling and needs assessment.

Mortality

It remains a paradox of health and social care needs assessment work that our most reliable source of data about the health of the population relates to data about deaths. Information about the numbers and causes of death are available for the UK and its constituent areas. Registration of death is compulsory and a doctor is required to certify the cause of death. The information that is recorded is as follows:

- date and place of death;
- name of deceased;
- sex of deceased;
- place of birth;
- date of birth;
- occupation;
- usual address.

The medical practitioner certifying the death is required to record the 'immediate' cause of death and then any underlying disease or condition which led to the death. The precision with which cause of death is identified varies considerably and is generally much less accurate for older people than those in younger age groups. It is almost inevitable that some causes of death which carry a considerable social stigma, such as AIDS, are under-reported.

Death registration data are collated and analysed by the ONS. Mortality statistics are presented in a variety of forms including the total numbers of deaths, geographical variations, causes of death and mortality rates. Data are published routinely for a variety of geographical areas such as counties or London boroughs.

The paucity of true morbidity measures has led many health service planners, those developing community care profiles and those responsible for resource allocation to use mortality statistics because of their ready availability. This is justified by the view that on the whole when mortality is high then so is morbidity, a view broadly confirmed by research studies. However, the usefulness of mortality data in developing community care based needs assessment is very limited. While current patterns of mortality may identify the areas or groups (such as older people) with poor health, such data may give a very poor picture of the present health risks and the possible need for community care. For example, data about the extent of mental health problems in the community are not well covered by mortality data. Mental illness is numerically a comparatively unimportant cause of death but is the cause of considerable morbidity and disability within the population. For example in 1992 in England and Wales 457 372 people aged 65 years of age and over died (this is 82% of all deaths) (OPCS, 1996). Of deaths amongst older people dementia accounted for 8417 deaths; 1.8% of all deaths among this age group. Similarly a needs assessment for those aged 65 years of age and over, based upon mortality data, would identify heart disease, cancer and respiratory disease as the main health problems while a morbidity based analysis would highlight the issue of osteo-arthritis, mental health problems and accidents (Victor, 1991).

Morbidity measures

Morbidity statistics are concerned with the amount and types of disability and illness that occur within the population. As such these would appear to be more appropriate measures to use in developing community care needs assessments. However, most of the morbidity data that are routinely collected suffer from serious shortcomings. This is partly due to of the variable nature and imprecise diagnosis of many illnesses, and partly because of inadequacies in the information system.

The main routinely available morbidity statistics are as follows:

- statutory notifications of infectious diseases;
- notification of episodes of sexually transmitted diseases;
- notification of 'prescribed' and other industrial disease and accidents;
- notification of congenital malformations;
- registration of handicapped persons;
- cancer registration.

As this list indicates, these data are only a very limited conceptualization of 'health' and are of little use in trying to develop a community care based needs assessment. Furthermore they are of little use in health based needs assessment because they are very dependent upon accurate identification and notification by medical practitioners. This probably means that, for some conditions, the notifications represent only a minority of the actual (or 'true') numbers of cases. Furthermore not all these data relate to individuals – some like the STD notifications relate to clinic attendances *not* individuals. Hence, routinely collected morbidity data are of no use in developing a community care based needs assessment for older people (although they may be of some use for other groups such as those with HIV/AIDs).

Surveys of health status and disability

Data about the overall health of the national population are available from several sources. First the 1991 censuses included a question about the number of individuals within households with 'long term limiting illness'. This is a very broad indicator of the prevalence of chronic health problems within the population. At both local and national level it correlates very well with data about mortality. As these data are available for small areas this measure may be a good way of identifying particular localities or districts that are experiencing health problems.

The General Household Survey (GHS), an annual social survey undertaken by ONS, collects data about the prevalence of both acute and chronic health problems as well as a variety of other topics. For a number of years (1980, 1985, 1991, 1994) they have included special sections on the difficulties that older people might have in managing the activities of daily living (such as mobility, self-care and housecare) which are essential for an independent life in the community. However, the GHS only includes within its study population those adults resident in the community. Excluded from the study are those resident in institutions (e.g. nursing and residential homes, prisons, etc.). This may limit the usefulness of the data it may provide when trying to profile the social care needs of older people.

ONS also sponsor a variety of *ad hoc* surveys looking at health issues. For example, they undertook a survey of the prevalence of disability within the population (Martin *et al.*, 1988) and in 1985 they undertook a special survey of carers as part of the General Household Survey (Green, 1988). They are often a useful source of broad prevalence rates which can then be applied to the particular context and can provide a broad indication of the scale of different problems within the communities served. Similarly, the English Health Survey can provide information about the health status of the population. However it has only a limited amount of information about disability issues. In order to use any of these data in local community care planning, it is necessary to apply national rates to the local population as these data are not available for local areas. For many health problems which may influence the need for community care, such as dementia or stroke, we often have to use data from locally based surveys or meta-analyses of such studies to arrive at an estimate of the number of people who may have reduced independence because of these problems. Furthermore almost all the data sources which are readily available relate to prevalence; comparatively little information is available about incidence.

FACTORS INFLUENCING THE NEED FOR COMMUNITY CARE

Arber and Ginn (1991) have argued that wellbeing in later life is dependent upon the inter-relationship between three aspects of life: access to caring resources, health and access to material resources. We would argue that these three aspects are all vital to any rigorous assessment of older peoples' needs for community care and we now consider each of these dimensions. Before this we will look at the demographic structure of the population and the key features of this which are relevant to community care.

Population composition

The age composition of the population is an important element in establishing the need for community care at a local (and indeed national level). Obviously, the number of older people (or the number of young adults or children) will influence the extent and type of demand for different community care services. In 1994 the estimated population of Great Britain was 53.3 million people of whom 20.6% (11.73 million people) were aged 60 years and over (Table 3.3). Nationally the percentage of the population aged 60 years and over shows some variation with the urban areas generally having a lower percentage of older people than the shire counties. In outer London 14.7% of the population are aged 65 years and over compared with 16.8% of the population of the shire counties and 15.7% nationally. This means that within each of the authorities responsible for providing community care there may be different levels of demand which need to be acknowledged in both the planning and funding of community care services.

Table 3.3 Great Britain: population by age and sex (000s)[a]

Age	Male	Female	Total	%
0–15	5871	5562	11 433	20.2
16–29	6013	5749	11 762	20.8
30–44	5984	5911	11 895	21.0
45–59	4769	4799	9568	16.9
60–74	3595	4185	7780	13.7
75–84	1914	1118	3032	5.3
85+	222	696	918	1.6
Total	27 571	28 817	56 388	99.5

[a]Derived from: OPCS, 1995b, Appendix 1

However, when we identify the population aged 60 years and over as 'older people' we are identifying a very large sub-group of the population as this can encompass a 60 years and over age-group. In particular, variations in the percentage of very elderly within a population can have an important influence upon the demand for care as this is the group which presents the highest prevalence of disability. Nationally, 1.6% of the population (or approximately 900 000 people) are aged 85 years or over and, again, there are local variations in both the number and percentage of older people who fall into this age group. When we identify the percentage of older people aged 85 years and over as a factor likely to influence the demand for community care we are using age as a proxy measure for need. As we will see in the sections on access to the different types of resources, not all very old people are frail or without resources. Therefore when developing population based assessments of community care needs we must be careful not to treat all older people (or all those aged 85 years and over) as an homogeneous group who will present identical needs.

Another factor that population based needs assessment must address is population change. The demographic structure of populations (be they countries or localities) are not static but are subject to change. Populations may grow or decline and the composition change. Community care plans must acknowledge the changing patterns of demand for their services and plan accordingly. Overall the national population is growing at a fairly slow rate. By the year 2001 it is estimated that the population of Great Britain will have increased by 7% (OPCS, 1995). However, some parts of the country are recording population decreases as people move out of the inner city districts.

Table 3.4 Great Britain: projections of the population aged 65 years and over, 1992–2021 (000s)[a]

Age (years)	1992	2001	2011	2021	% change 1991–2021
60–64	2798	2778	3725	3844	+37
65–69	2668	2495	2953	3219	+20
70–74	2317	2270	2320	3171	+36
75–79	1777	1908	1857	2272	+28
80–84	1255	1288	1398	1497	+19
85–89	649	772	876	919	+42
90+	269	439	562	672	+149

[a]Derived from: OPCS, 1995b, Appendix 1

The most significant feature of the population in the next decades is the ageing of the population (Victor, 1994). Over the 30 years 1991–2021, it is estimated that the population aged 60 years and over will increase by 32.9% (Table 3.4). This increase is not equally distributed across the age groups and is most pronounced among those people aged 85 and over. However the actual increases in the numbers in these age groups is rather less spectacular (e.g. the number of people aged 90 years and over will increase from 269 000 to 672 000). This is often referred to as 'the demographic timebomb' as it is thought to be accompanied by a decrease in the number of young people (though we should be cautious about this as it is notorious difficult to predict when and how many children each generation will produce).

While the increase in the numbers of older people is almost inevitable (as we are already born!), barring any major changes in mortality patterns, we cannot predict with any certainty what sorts of demands such groups may make upon the caring services. It is this large percentage increase in the numbers of the very elderly which provokes alarm because of:

- the greater prevalence of solo living amongst this group;
- the high levels of morbidity and disability among this population.

However, it is a matter of speculation as to whether future generations of older people will illustrate the same patterns of morbidity as today's cohorts of elders who have experienced considerable privation over their life course. Future generations of elders are likely to present a whole different set of needs because of the difference in experiences they will have had compared with the older people we see today.

The population aged 60 years and over is predominantly white with 3% of this age group identifying themselves as belonging to minority communities. In 1995 it is estimated that 20.9% of those who describe themselves as white were aged 60 years and over (CSO, 1996) compared with 5.8% of those from minority communities (7.2% black, 7.2% Indian, 4.3% Pakistani/Bangladeshi, 3.9% other). However, in the coming decades, we will see the 'ageing' of the minority communities which may well influence the nature of the demands for community care and the types and styles of services required.

Several other factors are important when assessing the need for community care – paramount among these are access to caring resources (e.g. household structure), health status and material circumstances. Each of these are now examined in turn.

Access to caring resources

In considering access to caring resources we need to distinguish between caring resources provided by the formal service sector (e.g. health services, private services) and those provided by the informal sector. Any comprehensive needs assessment must take stock of the formal resources which are available for caring for older people (or indeed other groups) within a defined locality. This means drawing together information about the activities of a whole variety of agencies. However it is important to remember that community care is supposed, in theory at least, to be a 'needs-led' policy. So, community care population level needs assessment should not be dominated by the current pattern of services provision. We will consider the contribution of the formal sector in caring for older people in Chapter 6.

Wenger (1984;1994) has clearly demonstrated that the social network available to older people is linked with their need for support from state services; those with wide social support networks are less likely to have to use state services than those with a very restricted network. However access to 'informal caring resources' is rather difficult to measure empirically and in a way which can be incorporated into a needs assessment. However routinely available data sources do provide information about two variables which may be taken as 'indirect' proxy measures of the availability of informal carers. These are marital status and household composition. To some extent these two variables are clearly interrelated. The household circumstances of older people obviously reflect the inter-relationship between age and civil status.

Table 3.5 describes the marital status of people aged 65 years and over. We can confine our attention to the situation in 1991 and see the often reported difference between older men and older women in their civil status. For men aged 65 years and over, three quarters are married compared with one-third of women. Almost half (49.2%) of the women are widowed. For women, the majority are widowed by the time they are aged 75–79 while for men the majority are not widowed until they are aged 90 years or over. Even in the very oldest age groups men are much more likely to be still married than women. This indicates that for old men they are likely to have a spouse to provide care while for women this is not the case.

Table 3.5 Marital status of those aged 65 years and over by age and sex (%): Great Britain 1991[a]

Age (years)	Single	Married	Divorced	Widowed
65–69				
m	8.1	78.6	4.1	9.2
f	7.2	58.6	4.7	29.6
70–74				
m	7.1	75.8	3.1	14.0
f	7.8	46.3	3.5	42.3
75–79				
m	6.7	69.2	2.3	21.8
f	9.2	32.4	2.5	55.9
80–84				
m	6.6	59.4	1.6	32.4
f	11.2	20.1	1.7	66.9
85–89				
m	6.7	46.6	1.2	45.5
f	13.2	11.1	1.2	74.5
90–94				
m	6.4	31.7	0.9	60.9
f	13.9	5.7	0.7	79.7
95–99				
m	6.6	20.5	1.1	71.8
f	15.4	3.5	0.5	80.6
100				
m	16.2	20.6	1.4	61.8
f	16.2	4.3	0.8	78.8

[a]Derived from: Jarvis *et al*, 1996

Table 3.6 Marital status of people aged 65 years and over (%): England and Wales 1971–2000[a]

	Single		Married		Divorced		Widowed	
	M	F	M	F	M	F	M	F
1971	7.0	14.2	72.7	35.3	0.6	0.7	19.4	49.5
1981	7.2	11.6	72.9	36.9	1.8	1.9	17.9	49.4
1991	6.9	8.8	72.3	38.3	3.2	3.5	16.8	49.2
2000[b]	8.0	7.0	69.0	39.0	5.0	6.0	18.0	49.0

[a]Derived from: OPCS, 1995b, Table 7
[b]Grundy, 1995, Table 6

Table 3.6 describes the civil status of people aged 65 years and more over the 20 year period 1971–1991. This table reveals that we cannot take distributions such as these as fixed and constant. Clearly illustrated is the demise of the spinsters. In 1971, 14% of women aged 65 years and over were classified as single (i.e. never married). This figure had almost halved by 1991 (8.8%), and decrease reflects an interesting cohort effect. The dying out of the group (or cohort) of now elderly women who had never married resulted from the lack of males in the wake of the devastation brought about by the 1914–1918 war. This serves to remind us that we cannot take for granted that the current civil status patterns will be shown by future generations of elders.

It seems almost inevitable that there will be an increase in the percentage of elderly people who are divorced and of those in second marriages. Indeed the table does hint at the increased prevalence of divorce among older people. It seems highly likely that future generations of elderly people will display more complicated household and family formation patterns as a result of these society changes. However, as we know so little of what marriage means to older people, it is difficult to predict what the effects of divorce and remarriage might be (see Askham, 1995).

Table 3.7 Household composition by age and sex (%): Great Britain 1994[a]

Household type	65–69		70–74		75–79		80–84		85+		All 65+	
	m	f	m	f	m	f	m	f	m	f	m	f
Alone	19	32	19	46	25	59	39	61	49	70	24	49
With spouse	63	51	66	40	62	28	50	20	41	10	47	35
With spouse+others	13	8	9	4	9	2	3	2	5	2	5	4
With siblings	1	1	3	2	1	3	3	4	1	3	2	2
With children	2	6	2	5	3	7	3	11	2	12	2	7
Other	1	2	1	2	1	1	1	2	1	3	1	2

[a]Derived from: GHS,1996,Table 6.3

Table 3.7 describes the household composition of older people and indicates that the majority live either alone or with their spouse. Only a minority of older people live in 'other' types of household such as with siblings or children. Again there is a very clear gender difference with older women much more likely to be living alone than their male contemporaries. Additionally, older women appear more likely to live with their children than do the men. Also, we need to recognize that there are variations between areas in the household circumstances of older people and that this will influence their needs for state care. In particular the prevalence of older people living alone is markedly higher in urban areas as compared with other parts of the country. It is especially high in inner London where 42% of those aged 65 years and over live alone. A more detailed description of the circumstances of older people in inner London is discussed elsewhere (Victor, 1996b).

Again the household circumstances of older people (and indeed other age groups) are not constant over time. The household situation of older people has changed markedly since 1945 when only 12% lived alone, which is only a marginal increase on the 7% reported for 1851 (Grundy, 1995). The increased prevalence of solo living is not confined to the older age groups but is a more general social trend. In 1961 14% of all households consisted of one person, compared with 27% in 1994/95 (CSO, 1996) and the number of households increased by 43% over this period (16.2 million to 23.1 million). Similarly, in 1961 4% of all households consisted of a single person under pensionable age and 7% were single people of pensionable age; by 1994/95 these percentages had increased to 12% and 15% respectively (CSO, 1996). Again it seems reasonable to expect that the percentage of older people living alone will increase in future decades and that this may result in further demands for social care, especially if family structures have been complicated and fragmented by the increased prevalence of divorce.

What are the wider family circumstances of older people and how much contact do they have with friends, relatives and neighbours? Data from the general household survey indicate that three quarters of those aged 65 years and over saw their relatives or friends weekly and the majority saw their neighbours for a chat (Table 3.8). However, levels of social contact are much lower among those in the oldest age groups. Of course we cannot infer from this that the friends, neighbours or relatives would be willing to contribute to the care of the older person simply because they are in contact with the older person. All these data do is indicate the social integration of the older people.

Table 3.8 Contact with neighbours and friends: population aged 65 years and over (%): Great Britain 1994[a]

Frequency of seeing friends/relatives	65–69		70–74		75–79		80–84		85+		All 65+	
	m	f	m	f	m	f	m	f	m	f	m	f
Daily	25	27	18	26	18	27	24	26	26	30	22	27
Weekly	51	53	52	56	53	53	52	51	48	53	52	52
Monthly	19	16	22	13	19	14	16	17	18	16	19	15
Less often	6	5	8	·4	10	7	8	6	7	9	7	6
At least weekly contact with neighbours	81	79	83	80	80	77	79	76	76	64	81	77

[a]Derived from: GHS, 1996, Tables 6.39 and 6.41

As we will see in Chapter 6, the family is a major source of care for older people. Apart from their spouse the next most important members of the caring network are sons and daughters (including in-laws). However it is not known how many older people have surviving children. Grundy (1995) estimates that, in 1962, 23% of those aged 65 years had no surviving children, 51% had one or two children and the rest had three or more children. She suggests that in 1986 slightly fewer older people had no surviving children (17%); 62% had one or two children and a much lower percentage had three or more children. This suggests that more older people had surviving children but that they had fewer numbers of children. This reflects the decrease in average family size which has taken place over the last 40 years. Of those with children, data from the British Social Attitudes Survey (Grundy, 1995) showed that for those aged 60 years or more, with sons and daughters, 12% saw their sons daily and 25% saw their daughter daily and that 70% and 80% respectively saw them monthly.

Health and disability

As has already been indicated the health status of older people is an important factor in enabling them to maintain an independent life in the community. Identifying the need for social and community care from health data is problematic for, as we have seen, few of the available indices relate to the ability of older people to live independently. In this context we are not, therefore interested in the prevalence (or incidence) of specific conditions such as hypertension or cancer, but rather on the effect of health conditions upon older people's ability to maintain their independence (for example the number of people left disabled after a stroke). However for some conditions such as stroke, dementia or arthritis we know that such conditions result in significant disability and a reduced ability of the older person to cope. Consequently data about the incidence and prevalence of such conditions can be applied to local populations and therefore can be useful in estimating needs for community care.

Dementia is a major source of disability within the community. However it is a relatively unimportant source of mortality accounting for 1.8% of deaths. Dementia is an important health problem which can result in a significant need for community care services (as well as health care services). Estimating the number of elderly people in the community suffering from dementia is problematic. It is particularly difficult to establish where along the continuum of behaviour that dementia starts. Jorm *et al.* (1987) have undertaken a meta-analysis of the various studies that have attempted to determine the prevalence (and incidence) of dementia in the community. Table 3.2, based upon the work of Jorm shows that the prevalence of clinically significant dementia (i.e. a degree of impairment of intellectual function which would merit service interventions by health and social service agencies) approximately doubles every five years; from 0.5% of those aged 60–64 years to 34% of those aged 90 years and over. Applying these to the population of Great Britain implies that there are 707 897 people aged 60 years and over with this condition (approximately 6% of the population). Numerically, the largest number of people with dementia is to be found among those aged 80–84 years. Table 3.2 indicates that, unless there is a significant change in the natural history of this disease, there will be a 32% increase in the number of people with dementia and that the largest number of cases will be found among the very old (i.e. those aged 90 years and over).

The above data relate to the prevalence of the condition. However, it is also useful to know the incidence of the condition. How many new cases are diagnosed each year? Brayne and Ames (1988) suggest we should use the guestimate of 1% per annum for the population aged 65 years and over. This suggests that, in Great Britain, there are 90 650 new clinically significant cases of dementia annually.

The General Household Survey is an annual survey of the population living in the community, which has been running since 1972. In 1980, 1985, 1991 and 1994 they have asked those people aged 65 years and over about their ability to undertake various activities of daily living. These supplementary questions relate directly to the ability of older people to live independently in the community. Although the exact questions asked have varied each year they have broadly covered three aspects of daily life. These are; mobility, self-care (such as dressing and feeding) and domestic care tasks (such as shopping, cooking and cleaning). There have been no significant changes in the percentages of those people able to undertake these activities over the time period covered by the GHS (Table 3.9). We may assume, therefore, for the present that we are unlikely to see significant changes in the percentages of older people unable to manage these types of activities.

Table 3.9 Percentage of those aged 65 years and over unable to manage selected activities of daily living: Great Britain 1980–1994[a]

	1980	1985	1991	1994
Going outdoors and walking down road	12	13	11	13
Getting up/down steps and stairs	8	9	9	9
Getting around house on level	2	2	2	1
Getting to the toilet	2	2	1	1
Getting in/out of bed	2	2	2	2
Wash face and hands	1	1	1	0
Feed self	0	1	1	0
Household shopping	14	16	19	16
Clean windows inside	17	19	16	20
Wash clothes by hand	7	8	8	7

[a]Derived from: Goddard and Savage, 1994, Tables 29, 32, 39; GHS, 1996, Tables 6.24 and 6.32

The activities of daily living are divided into three main categories: mobility, self care and domestic tasks (Tables 3.10–3.12). With each category the percentage unable to manage these tasks increases with age. Highlighting those aged 85 years and over, these tables reveal that at least 20% are unable to manage one of the self-care tasks, 60% cannot manage household shopping, 51% cannot clean windows and 44% have at least one mobility problem.

Table 3.10 Percentage unable to undertake locomotion activities of daily living on own: Great Britain 1994[a]

	65–69	70–74	75–79	80–84	85+	All 65+
Going out or walking down road	7	8	13	21	37	13
Getting up/down steps	6	7	8	13	23	9
Getting around house	1	1	0	2	3	1
Getting to the toilet	2	1	0	2	3	1
Getting in/out of bed	2	2	1	2	4	2

[a]Derived from: GHS, 1996, Table 6.22

Table 3.11 Percentage those aged 65 years and over unable to undertake self-care tasks: Great Britain 1994[a]

	65–69	70–74	75–79	80–84	85+	All 65+
Wash all over	4	6	8	14	21	8
Dress/undress	2	3	2	4	6	3
Wash face/hands	0	1	0	0	1	0
Feeding	1	0	0	0	1	0
Cut toenails	16	25	34	54	60	31

[a]Derived from: GHS, 1996, Table 6.28

Table 3.12 Percentage those aged 65 years and over unable to undertake domestic tasks: Great Britain 1994[a]

	65–69	70–74	75–79	80–84	85+	All 65+
Household shopping	8	11	17	26	47	16
Wash/dry dishes	2	2	2	2	6	2
Clean inside windows	11	13	22	30	53	20
Use vacuum	6	6	9	15	30	10
Wash clothes by hand	4	6	7	10	14	7
Cook main meal	2	4	5	8	15	5
Prepare snack	1	2	1	3	7	2
Make a cup of tea	1	1	1	2	5	1

[a]Derived from: GHS, 1996, Tables 6.30 and 6.33

Application of prevalence estimates to local populations is a powerful way of expressing the potential need for services within communities. The large numbers of people within a locality who are likely to experience such problems is illustrated by Table 3.13. In this table, the prevalence of older people unable to manage selected activities of daily living and of those with dementia have been applied to the population of Surrey. This illustrates the sheer scale of the potential numbers of people who may need community care within a locality. For example, there were 8822 people unable to wash, and there would be 1700 new cases of dementia annually. Given funding limitations, it is highly unlikely that all these needs could be met if they were presented to the local authority.

Table 3.13 Estimated numbers of those aged 65 years and over unable to manage selected activities of daily living in Surrey[a]

	Prevalence rate (%)	Estimated number in Surrey
Unable to manage steps/stairs	9	15 880
Unable to get in/out of bed	2	3529
Unable to wash all over	8	8822
Unable to dress	3	7057
Unable to feed	1	1764
Unable to shop	16	33 524
Unable to use vacuum cleaner	10	19 409
Unable to cook main meal	5	10 587
With clinically significant dementia	3–5	5293–10 587

[a]Surrey had an estimated population of 10 397 000 in 30/6/93 of whom 176 443 were aged 65 years and over

In developing a population based needs assessment for community care the OPCS disability survey is an important source of data (Martin *et al.* 1988). This survey attempted to estimate the causes of disability within the population (both those resident in the community and those living in institutions) and the severity of disability within the population. The study included both adults and children and those living in institutions as well as those in the community. For the purpose of community care profiling only the community based prevalence estimates should be used.

Table 3.14 The prevalence of different types of disability in the community: Great Britain 1996[a]

	Rate per 1000		Estimated numbers	
	60–74	75+	60–74	75+
Locomotion	195	464	1 487 850	1 918 640
Reaching/stretching	52	129	396 760	533 415
Dexterity	76	180	579 880	744 300
Sight	52	225	396 760	930 375
Hearing	108	307	824 040	1 269 445
Personal care	93	263	709 590	1 087 505
Continence	38	120	289 940	496 200
Communication	38	112	289 940	463 120
Behaviour	36	88	274 680	363 880
Intellectual function	37	107	282 310	442 445
Consciousness	4	6	30 520	24 810
Feeding	11	18	83 930	74 430
Disfigurement	18	27	137 340	111 645

[a]Derived from: Martin *et al.*, 1988, Table 3.13

Table 3.14 presents the prevalence rate for different types of disability. Problems with mobility are the most common type of disability experienced by older people. However, these data indicate that, in the community, there are 1 087 505 people aged 75 years and over who have problems with personal care, about half a million (496 200) with continence problems and 442 445 with impaired intellectual functions.

However, while identifying the types of disability in the community these data do not enlighten us as to the severity of the disability. For example, difficulties with personal care could range from difficulties putting on socks and shoes to a complete inability to dress oneself. Consequently, Table 3.15 shows the prevalence of the 10 point disability scale developed by OPCS. Rather than consider each point on the disability scale, it is more useful to develop categories that relate to the need for community care. The DoH (1993) describe a three point scale which relates to community care needs. High need (9, 10 on the severity scale) describes those who need help on a daily basis, moderate need describes those who need help several times a week (but not daily) and low need identifies potentially frail people who may need 'preventive' help. Table 3.16 presents the prevalence rates for these three categories and indicates that 367 918 people aged over 60 years would be classified as being in high need (54% of whom were aged 80 years).

Table 3.15 Prevalence of different disability in the community by severity levels: Great Britain, 1996[a]

Category	Rate per 1000		
	60–69	70–79	80+
10 (worst)	3	6	25
9	10	17	60
8	11	23	57
7	14	28	60
6	15	37	69
5	27	44	86
4	28	45	68
3	31	53	71
2	41	65	68
1 (best)	56	77	90

[a]Derived from: Martin *et al.*, 1988, Table 3.4

Table 3.16 Estimated numbers of disabled people in the community : Great Britain, 1996

Severity category	Rate per 1000			Estimated numbers		
	60–69	70–79	80+	60–69	70–79	80+
High (9–10)	13	24	85	68 601	99 312	200 005
Moderate (4–8)	95	177	340	501 315	732 426	800 020
Low (1–3)	128	195	229	675 456	806 910	538 837

Access to material resources

The final element of a population based community care needs assessment for older people is concerned with access to material resources. In this section we will consider the financial circumstances and housing of older people as these are directly related to the older persons ability to pay for care.

Only a small percentage of those people aged 60–65 years and over, 13%, are still in paid employment. Therefore, job-related earnings are a comparatively unimportant element of pensioners incomes. Consequently older people are dependent upon three main sources for their income: state benefits/pensions (received by about 98% of older people), private (occupational) pensions (received by 53% of older people) and income from savings and investments (received by 65% of older people) (Victor, 1996a).

There has been much discussion about the financial circumstances of older people (Johnson and Falkingham, 1992). In particular it was suggested that older people were improving their financial circumstances relative to other sectors of the population. This was true only in relation to other groups who were also dependent on benefit such as the long-term unemployed (Falkingham and Victor, 1991). The gulf between older people and the rest of the employed population remains large with only a few very well off older people (the so-called woopies) (Falkingham and Victor, 1991). Victor 1996a reports that only 7% of people aged 65 years and over are in the top 20% of the income distribution compared with 39% in the bottom 20%. Overall, it is estimated that 60% of pensioners' income is derived from the state, 20% from occupational pensions, 14% from savings/investments and 6% from earnings (Victor, 1996a). The relative importance of state and non-state sources of income varies within the elderly population. It is only among the younger components of the population at the top of the income distribution where non-state sources of income are of major significance (Victor, 1996a; Hancock and Weir, 1994). Women, those living alone, those over 80 years of age and those from a background of unskilled manual jobs are those most at risk of experiencing poverty and low income in later life (Victor, 1996a; Arber and Ginn, 1991; Johnson and Falkingham, 1992, Townsend, 1979). It is precisely those sectors of the older population experiencing the greatest health needs, who have the least access to household caring resources and who have least ability to pay for the care they need. Groves (1995) concludes that, on the basis of current research evidence, only a small minority of older people can realistically make a significant contribution towards the cost of community care.

Housing is another factor that is an important element in the material resources available to older people. This is for two main reasons: first, the home provides the location within which older people live, and it has a very important meaning for older people (and indeed other age groups). Second, the quality, design and state of repair of the dwelling can obviously hinder (or promote) the ability of older people to live independently. Finally for those who are home owners, this represents a significant financial asset which could, in theory at least, be released to provide resources to contribute to the care of the older person. In 1994, 55% of those aged 65 years and over owned their home outright while another 9% had an outstanding mortgage, compared with 42% and 5% respectively in 1980 (Jarvis *et al.*, 1996). Over the same period renting from the council decreased from 41% to 30% and private renting from 12% to 6% (Jarvis *et al.*, 1996).

The prevalence of home ownership is highest among the 'younger' elderly, with 72% of those aged 60–64 years classed as home owners compared with 57% of those aged 80 years and over. So, it is precisely those who are most in need of care who are least likely to be home owners. Hamnett (1995) suggests that it is highly unlikely that anything other than a minority of older people will use their houses to fund care especially as this is in direct opposition to the stated policy objective of allowing wealth to trickle down between the generations.

Most older people remain in their own homes during their later life. However 10% of those aged 65 years and over live in sheltered accommodation (GHS, 1996). This percentage ranges from 7% of those aged 65–69 years to 18% of those aged 85 years and over (GHS, 1996).

CONCLUSION

In this chapter we have examined some of the methodological issues which need to be considered when undertaking population level needs assessment for community care for older people (and indeed other age groups). In addition we have examined the main substantive factors which are likely to influence both national and local demands for community care by older people. However, population level needs assessment is only the first element in developing community care. In the next chapter we will examine the issues underlying the assessment of need at the individual level.

Assessment of individual needs   4

INTRODUCTION

Perhaps the defining element of the community care changes is the notion that services which are provided out of public funds should only be given after a thorough review (or assessment) of the individual. The NHS and Community Care Act (NHSCCA, 1990) made the assessment of need for 'community care services' a duty for local authorities. After an assessment, they must then decide if services should be provided. The NHSCCA (sections 47, (1a) and (1b) describe this as follows: 'any person for whom they may provide or arrange for the provision of community care services may be in need of any such services'. The authority must carry out an assessment of needs for services and decide whether these needs call for provision of such services. The assessment is used both to ensure that entry to publicly funded long-term care is based upon 'need' and to identify those individuals who can best be supported in their own homes.

According to Leicester and Pollock (1996), older people now face three barriers which they must overcome if they are to be successful recipients of community care. First, they must show that they are eligible to have their needs assessed (i.e. they must fulfil the appropriate eligibility criteria). Second they must demonstrate their eligibility for services through the assessment of their needs and finally they may have to undergo a financial assessment (or means test) to see if they must contribute towards any services that they receive. Each of these issues are considered in detail in this chapter.

The White Paper (DoH, 1989) offers some indication as to how the assessment of individually based needs should be undertaken. It states that the local authority has a duty to assess those individuals needing 'social care and support e.g. for mobility, personal care, domestic tasks, financial offers, accommodation, leisure and employment, which they cannot arrange for themselves' (DoH, 1989, para. 3.2.2.). It is further stated that 'Assessment should take into account the wishes of the individual and his or her carer, and of the carer's ability to continue to provide care ... efforts should be made to offer flexible services which enable individuals and carers to make choices' (DoH, 1989, para. 3.2.6).

WHO IS ELIGIBLE FOR COMMUNITY CARE?

In the original legislation, assessments were for the person who was asking for support. As noted above, the assessment should take into account the wishes of carers but these were seen as secondary to those of the applicant. However, carers are now entitled to an assessment for community care needs in their own right following The Carers (Recognition and Service) Act (1995) which came into force in April 1996. However, assessment does not mean that it automatically follows that people will be provided with services.

Who, then, is eligible for community care? There is little in The White Paper (DoH, 1989) and subsequent Parliamentary Act as to who is (and who is not) eligible for assessment for community care. It is stated that people 'who appear to need community care services' are those who are eligible for assessment. Clearly this is a very loose and ill-defined term which is open to a myriad of interpretations. There is no other more specific guidance upon eligibility for assessment (and it is to be remembered that assessment does not necessarily result in the provision of services). Hence, in the absence of central guidance local variation is going to be an integral part of the way that community care is implemented in Britain.

Each local authority must publish information about the criteria they use to establish individuals' eligibility for assessment. In theory these are supposed to be expressed in terms of eligibility needs for assistance and set in order of priority. Central government states that these criteria should be drawn up in consultation with health agencies, housing authorities and other service providers. Criteria should also include details of how to apply for an assessment, eligibility for assessment, how eligibility is decided, how to complain and details of services provided. Such information should be available to all who need it (e.g. non English speakers or those with communication difficulties). A social services inspectorate study of five social service departments for the year 1993/94 concluded that the sample authorities had made considerable progress in making information about eligibility criteria and the assessment process widely available (SSI, 1994). However, the presentation of such material was not always as 'user friendly' as the spirit of the community care changes might have hoped. Furthermore, it is not clear how the material has been received by (potential) users and carers.

There have been few systematic studies of the eligibility criteria used by local authorities. Indeed, a study by the Association of County Councils/Association of Metropolitan Authorities (ACC/AMA) (1995) commented that in their study they could not undertake any systematic review of eligibility criteria because of the highly disparate nature of the material they were trying to summarize.

Leicester (1994) looked at eligibility criteria in the eight local authorities in the former South West Thames Regional Health Authority (RHA). She reported that four local authorities had published clear definitions of high, low and moderate need. Information is also presented as to the definitions used in Barking and Dagenham (DoH, 1993). Table 4.1 indicates that there is considerable degree of agreement between the four authorities as to what defines 'high' need. In Surrey and Barking the definitions of need relate to the categories used in the OPCS disability survey (Martin *et al.*, 1988). Elsewhere, the definitions of high need in the other areas appear difficult to quantify. Hence most authorities using these types of statements could neither estimate the number of individuals in each category within their area nor the impact that this would have upon services. However for both Surrey and Barking the number of older people in each category may be estimated, thereby providing some understanding of potential demand and the prevalence rates for these different need categories (Table 3.16; chapter 3).

Table 4.1 Eligibility criteria: definitions of 'high need'[a]

Barking and Dagenham: people who need help with personal care tasks every day (e.g. people who, without help, are unable to get in/out of bed, eat and drink, get to and use wc/commode, wash hands and face) and/or are incontinent, mentally infirm (this approximates to people in categories 9, 10 of the OPCS disability scale).

Surrey: people who need assistance every day with getting in/out of bed, eating and drinking, preparing light snacks, getting to and using wc/commode, getting dressed, washing face and hands, and who may be incontinent and/or mentally infirm. Also people who would not be able to function safely or lead independent lives unless they received the provision of adaptations or equipment.

Richmond: people who need frequent assistance throughout the day with personal care tasks including: getting in/out of bed, bathing and washing hands/face, using the wc/commode, assistance in maintaining continence, getting dressed, eating and drinking. Also people with the following problems: dementia or disorientation, severely restricted.

Kingstown: people who, without assistance, would not be able to undertake the following activities of daily living: personal care tasks (such as washing, dressing, getting up/going to bed, assistance with medication) and practical tasks (such as shopping, domestic cleaning, payment of bills, pension collection).

Croydon: as for Surrey plus those at serious risk due to mental and/or physical frailty e.g. falling, wandering etc. and/or due to physical, emotional or financial abuse.

[a]Derived from: Leicester and Pollock, 1996, Table 2; DoH, 1993

There was less agreement as to what constituted moderate and low need (Tables 4.2 and 4.3). For example, in Richmond a person needing help three times a week is defined as being in 'low' need whereas they would be defined as being in moderate need by Surrey and Croydon. Leicester (1994) observes that there was uncertainly as to the 'meaning' of these needs criteria. Did they describe eligibility for assessment, eligibility of services or simply some indication of different levels of need? There was, at the time this work was undertaken, variation between the four authorities in receipt of services. One authority only provided services for those in the high need category while others still provided care to those in the moderate or low need categories. However given the financial pressure that local authorities are under it seems increasingly likely that services will be targeted at those in greatest need. In terms of helping older people to remain in the community, this may not be the most effective option. We might speculate that there is little that could be done to prevent long-term care admission for the most disabled. However it could be that services might be most effectively used by those in the 'moderate' need group and for whom prevention of long-term care admission might be a realistic objective. In the absence of rigorous evaluation data this must remain pure speculation.

Table 4.2 Eligibility criteria: definitions of 'moderate need'[a]

Barking and Dagenham: people who need assistance several times a week but less than daily (with bathing/strip washing, shopping, light household cleaning, cooking meals) and/or are mildly confused (this approximates to a score of 4–8 on the OPCS disability scale).

Surrey: need assistance several times a week to: bath/strip wash, do shopping, light household cleaning, cook meals and/or are mildly confused.

Richmond: people who need assistance on a daily basis with the following tasks: preparation of light snacks, getting dressed. Also people with mild confusion/disorientation.

Kingston: people who retain some capacity to undertake daily living tasks but who need assistance to maintain their level of functioning. This will include people with severe disabilities who are able to undertake most personal care but need assistance with practical tasks such as cleaning, meal preparation and some personal tasks such as bathing and hair washing.

Croydon: same as Surrey plus people who require assistance or support due to social isolation/lack of motivation or due to the stresses of caring relationships.

---

[a]Derived from: Leicester and Pollock, 1996, Table 2; DoH, 1993

Table 4.3 Eligibility criteria: definitions of 'low need'[a]

Barking and Dagenham: potentially frail people who may need some preventative services (e.g. people who have some disability but do not need help more than once a week).

Surrey: as Barking and Dagenham.

Richmond: people who need assistance with some or all of the following tasks at least three times a week: bathing/strip washing, preparation of meals, household cleaning, shopping, important visits (e.g. dentist).

Kingston: people who are able to care for themselves but who, because of physical impairment or mental problems, will benefit from assistance with tasks such as pension collection, cleaning, shopping or getting in/out the bath.

Croydon: as Barking and Dagenham.

---

[a]Derived from: Leicester and Pollock, 1996, Table 2; DoH, 1993

The framework of the legislation concerning eligibility criteria raises two important points. There are no nationally agreed eligibility criteria for assessments of care needs and no nationally agreed method for assessing care needs. Furthermore, there are, with the exception of residential and nursing home care, no standard procedures for changing. Consequently, community care in all its aspects will show variation between different parts of the country. Indeed variation between local authority areas is encouraged. This contrasts with the underlying founding philosophy of the NHS which was to create equality of access to health care irrespective of any factor (e.g. social class, geographical location) other than need. However with the changes to the NHS, included in the 1991 Act, this too is moving to a less homogenous (and possibly less equitable) mode of provision. We will return to the issue of eligibility for different types of services in Chapters 5 and 7.

RELATING INDIVIDUAL AND POPULATION LEVEL NEEDS ASSESSMENT

We have already seen that population level needs assessment is an important aspect of the implementation of community care. Individual assessments are also important. However, these are not undertaken in a vacuum as there is a clear link between the two activities which should increase over time. Initial population level assessments are likely to be undertaken using the types of data described in Chapter 3. However, in theory at least, the results of individual assessments can be collated and aggregated to present a picture of the actual needs presented. This, of course, requires a considerable degree of information sharing within an agency and the development of assessment schedules suitable for turning into aggregate indices. A comprehensive computing system is also required, and it is unclear as to how many local authorities have such an infrastructure.

These data can then be compared with the theoretical needs derived from the population perspective and any discrepancies reviewed. For example, a lower than projected level of assessments may reflect the availability of a comprehensive and robust informal caring network or the failure of older people to come forward and ask for help. Clearly, local research may be required to examine any observed differences. Theoretical comparisons could be made between areas in the levels and types of assessments being made. However the enormous variability between areas in the nature and content of the assessment process makes this virtually impossible.

Types of assessment

The Practitioners Guide (DoH, 1991a, para. 3.3) describes the assessment process thus: 'the assessment process should be as speedy, simple and as informal as possible ... based on the principle of what is the least that it is necessary to know to understand the needs being presented and to justify the investment of public resources'. However, assessing needs at the level of the individual can be every bit as complex as population based needs assessment. The impression given in the policy guidance accompanying the White Paper presents the issue of assessment as uncontentious and unproblematic both conceptually and practically. There are two important issues regarding assessment which need to be resolved before it can be successfully implemented; what 'level' of assessment is required to meet the needs presented and how should the assessment be conducted (this relates to both the substance of the assessment and the way that it is structured and administered). Each of these are now considered in turn.

As indicated above, it is intended that the assessment process should be speedy. However it is clear that, at the most basic level, older people may present a variety of needs ranging from the straightforward to the highly complex. Some needs can be identified and solved using a fairly simple and straightforward assessment while others are likely to be much more complex. Consequently six potential levels of assessment are described in the Practitioners Guide. These range from the simple which are usually for a single need (e.g. a request for a travel pass), through limited assessment to comprehensive assessments for individuals with complex needs which carry a high level of risk and which require multi-agency multi-service response.

The graded levels of assessment were proposed to cope with the varying levels of complexity of individuals' needs. However this is a very complicated scheme and, more fundamentally, it is difficult to see how the correct grade of assessment can be given before identification of the individuals needs. For example, it is difficult to see how a practitioner could decide between a limited assessment (limited, defined needs and low risk) and a multiple assessment (range of limited, defined, low risk needs) without having undertaken a needs assessment. Clearly, this number of levels of assessment would be very difficult to operationalize.

The Audit Commission (1992) recognized these problems and prosposed an alternative model which could respond to the variety of individual needs presented and relate to the policies and eligibility criteria set at a strategic level by individual local authorities. The Audit Commission's model was based upon a system of assessment used in the London Borough of Islington and consisted of three levels; a screening level, a simple level and a complex level. According to Meredith (1995), most authorities have asked for three levels of assessment, simple, specialist and comprehensive. Decisions have to be made for individuals as to what level of assessment is appropriate and this is sometimes termed 'screening'.

Some examples of the assessment process

Leicester (1994) documented the assessment process in the eight local authority areas (Croydon, Kingston, Merton, Richmond, Sutton, Wandsworth and Surrey) which were within the former South West Thames RHA. These eight local authorities illustrated considerable diversity in the way they have structured the assessment process. Indeed, it is sometimes rather difficult to discern from the documentation how the assessment process actually works.

Table 4.4 Summary of assessment process in eight local authorities in former South West Thames RHA[a]

Local Authority	Assessment process
Croydon	level 1 – preliminary assessment – checks against eligibility
	level 2 – simple need
	level 3 – complex assessment
Kingston	initial request
	single service need
	wide ranging need
Merton	simple request (e.g. bus pass)
	single source need = standard assessment
	more complex need = enhanced assessment
	complex assessment = multidisciplinary assessment
Richmond	initial enquiry – checks against eligibility criteria
	care assessment
	comprehensive assessment
Surrey	screening assessment – checks against targeting criteria
	formal assessment
Sutton	simple care assessment
	comprehensive assessment if meet criteria
Wandsworth	checks against eligibility criteria
	assessment of need
West Sussex	simple needs
	detailed needs

[a]Derived from: Leicester, 1994

We will return to the substantive issue of assessments and the experience of assessment later in this chapter. Here we will confine our attention to the consideration of how the system works. In four of the local authority areas (Croydon, Surrey, Wandsworth and Richmond) a preliminary assessment is made at the point of referral (Table 4.4). If individuals do not meet the targeting/eligibility criteria they are given advice and referred elsewhere (e.g. to a voluntary or self-help agency). In five of the local authorities (West Sussex, Wandsworth, Surrey, Sutton and Richmond) there are two types of assessment; simple and complex. In simple assessment there is usually a single, well defined problem which results in a fairly simple service response from a single agency e.g. provision of home help. Complex assessments are those with a more intricate pattern of needs which require intensive levels of service provision and usually necessitate a multi-agency multi-disciplinary response. Hence, in practice the levels of assessment being offered to older people are much more straightforward and less complex than perhaps originally intended. It is evident that each local authority has attempted to follow DoH guidelines and to distinguish between the assessments at different levels of complexity. However no authority has tried to operate the original six levels of assessment. Instead, they have opted for a two-stage approach. Based upon the above data, Figure 4.1 presents an overview of the type of two-stage assessment process which seems to be most common in the former South

West Thames RHA. Similar trends have been reported nationally (DoH, 1993). However the effectiveness of this pattern of assessments (or indeed any other) has not been rigorously evaluated. Hence, decisions about the 'best' way of implementing this aspect of community care are being made locally and based on experience, custom and practice.

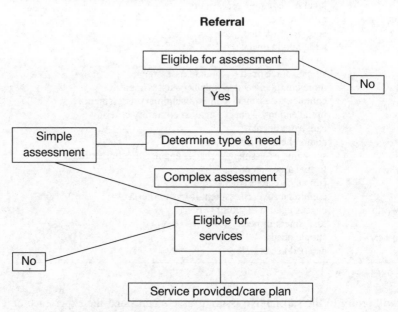

Figure 4.1 Simplified outline of two-stage assessment process

Individual assessment: What is 'need'?

The DoH (1991a) in the Practitioners Guide, state that it is essential that all agencies and people involved in community care share a common understanding of the term 'need'. While this seems to make good sense, it is very difficult to achieve in practice as this is a term which has a plethora of different meanings. It goes on to define need as 'the requirements of individuals to enable them to achieve, maintain or restore an acceptable level of social independence or quality of life, *as defined by the particular care agency* (my emphasis)'. Thus, although the philosophy of the community care changes is that of providing needs-led services it is not a user-led service. In the last instance, needs are endorsed (or rejected) by those undertaking the assessment and not by those who are assessed. This is emphasized again by the Practitioners Guide (DoH, 1991a) which states quite explicitly that '… having weighted the views of all parties, including his/her own observation, the assessing practitioner is responsible for defining the user's needs' (DoH, 1991a, para. 3.5).

What should be included in an assessment of needs?

The above definition of need relates to two issues; social independence and quality of life. However to undertake any form of needs assessment we need to turn these rather general and ill-defined notions into concepts, which can be used when collecting information from individuals who are undergoing an assessment. Initially, the guidance for managers which accompanied the community care changes (DoH, 1991b) described six dimensions which should be included in the assessment of individual need. These were:

- personal/social care;
- health care;
- accommodation;
- finance;
- education/employment/leisure;
- transport/access.

Table 4.5 Areas of need suggested for inclusion in a comprehensive assessment[a]

Areas of need	Standardized instruments available
Biographical details	No
Self perceived needs	No
Self care	Yes
Physical health	Yes
Mental health	Yes
Use of medicines	Yes
Abilities, attitudes and lifestyle	No
Race and culture	No
Personal history	No
Needs of carers	Yes
Social network and support	Yes
Care services	Yes
Housing	No
Transport	No
Risk	No
Finance	No

[a]Derived from: DoH, 1991b

These categories were expanded in the Practitioners Guide (DoH, 1991a) to form the 16 categories shown in Table 4.5. There are clearly some direct overlaps between these two lists, such as accommodation and finance. However, the expanded list contains some important areas excluded from the original guidance such as carers' needs. Nevertheless, scrutiny of the variables which it is suggested should be used to record these different domains reveals some important omissions. For example, postcode which is a key variable for developing population based needs assessment is not included and neither is the current location of the client (e.g. home, relatives homes, etc.). As this is conceptualized it gives the appearance of a static single point in time assessment, but it does appear to take heed of changes in older people's lives such as bereavement or changes in place of residence. Within the list of self-care tasks there is a heavy concentration upon 'female' tasks such as cooking and shopping but no mention of important tasks such as household repairs or gardening.

More fundamentally there are a variety of standardized measures available for measuring some of the categories such as self-care needs but none of these are recommended by the DoH for inclusion in the assessment. This is a fundamental weakness of the assessment process, and it makes comparison between areas and with population data available from elsewhere (e.g. the GHS) impossible. This is not a feature unique to the field of community care. For example, although the DoH prescribes the areas which must be included in the over 75s screening which GPs undertake, it declines to indicate how these should be conducted and how the various aspects of life should be measured. This makes a potentially useful source of data about the health (and to some extent social care) needs of older people useless for the development of services, and it is of little value for research. We will return to the issue of using standardized assessment schedules in needs assessments later in this chapter.

Table 4.6 Models of topics for inclusion in a comprehensive assessment

Hughes (1995)	Payne (1993)
Attitude to self	
Physical health	Health and capacity
	Oppression/abuse
Functioning	Education/retirement activity
Personal characteristics	
Family/support networks	Relationships
Community relationships	
Environment	Housing/environment
Financial/material	Employment
Circumstances	
Recreational activities	Leisure/social stimulation

Views upon which aspects of older people's lives are included within the comprehensive assessment are not confined to central government. Hughes (1995) and Payne (1993) have suggested alternative models identifying topics that they think should be covered (Table 4.6). There are some overlaps (such as all three models agree that health should be recorded) but there is also considerable diversity as to what should be included/excluded. This serves to highlight that there is no 'agreed' consensus about which topic areas assessment should cover.

THE ASSESSMENT OF OLDER PEOPLE

Assessment is the cornerstone of community care. It operates at both individual and population levels. One important factor which will impact upon how well (or otherwise) the community care changes operate is the way individuals are assessed – what information is collected and how it is collected. This will effect both the individual needs assessment and the development of population profiles derived from the aggregation of individual assessments. One way in which the latter part of this process could be made more rigorous is by using standardized assessment schedules (or instruments) rather than locally designed measures.

The ways in which the DoH suggests there should be coverage of a complex assessment of an individual's needs have been described. In this section, we will discuss some of the methodological issues underpinning assessment and consider which of these should be involved in the development of such tools.

There are a wide variety of assessment instruments available for use with older people (Fletcher, 1994). Within the health care context these types of standardized schedules are often termed 'outcome measures'. As such, these instruments are usually designed in order to be able to evaluate the extent to which a health care intervention has achieved its desired outcome (e.g. does treatment in a stroke unit decrease mortality, decrease disability and increase quality of life). Jinkinson (1994) reviews the development of health outcome measures, and Victor (1996b) discusses the problems in applying these to older populations.

These health outcome type measures have been designed to consider various aspects of older people's lives in a variety of different settings (e.g. home, hospital or primary care). Measures are available to assess the performance of older people in all the main areas of daily living including physical health (e.g. mobility and personal care), mental health (e.g. memory, behaviour and emotional), social support and social networks. Indeed the Royal College of Physicians (RCP)/British Geriatrics Society (BGS) (1992) have recommended a set of standardized instruments which should be used in assessing the health related needs of older people. These are listed in Table 4.7 and clearly link with some of the areas which the DoH has suggested should be included in a complex community care assessment. As there are a variety of texts which describe the available measures we will not examine these here (Bowling, 1995; 1991).

Table 4.7 Scales recommended for use with older people[a]

Activities of daily living	Barthel scale
Cognitive function	Abbreviated mental test score
Depression	Geriatric depression scale
Quality of life	Philadelphia geriatric centre Morale scale

[a]Derived from: RCP/BGS, 1992

What are the main methodological and practical issues underlying the choice of any assessment instruments. These relate to two main aspects; the design of the schedule and the scientific rigour of the measures used. These are now considered in turn. For those who are not involved in the design of assessment schedules, a knowledge of these aspects will enable them to be more critical of the results of such assessments.

Technical considerations in choosing assessment instruments

As we have seen, the term 'assessment' is widely used and, as such, has come to mean different things to different people. Fletcher (1994) notes that assessment measures of elderly people is generally used in one (or more) of the following contexts:

- screening – this is to identity individuals in need of further assessment;
- management of individuals – in this situation the instrument is used as a diagnostic aid and a way of setting individual goals;
- descriptive studies – specific instruments may be used to profile the main characteristics of certain populations of older people;
- evaluation of health services or interventions (e.g. the use by Vetter *et al.* of the Townsend disability index (1984));
- audit – to monitor the quality of care delivered to specific patient populations. A set of instruments for use with elderly people has been drawn up (RCP/BGS, 1992).

It is important to note that none of the standardized instruments has been developed for the purpose of identifying specific needs at the individual level. However they do have the merit of being building blocks for developing community profiles and for enabling comparisons between areas.

How should assessments be conducted?

Before discussing the ideal technical properties of assessment schedules, it is necessary to consider the practicalities of how assessment data are to be collected. Assessments may be carried out in a variety of different settings including the older person's own home, hospital or elsewhere, and they may take place over a series of days. These constraints will influence the way the schedule is designed.

In designing any assessment tool it is important to consider the following technical issues.

- How do the instruments work (are they self completion questionnaires or interviewer administered, are they 'paper and pencil' forms or entered directly onto a computer)?
- How long do the assessments take to complete?
- Are the questions acceptable to users?

- What format do the questions take (e.g. closed questions with a predetermined set of answers (which is very suited to computerization and aggregate analysis) or open questions where individuals can express themselves in their own words).

The community care changes have generated large numbers of assessments. For example, Leicester (1994) estimates that, in the London Borough of Wandsworth, there are 4000 assessments per year of which 74% are accounted for by people aged 65 years and over. Given the large numbers of assessments involved it is imperative, from the local authorities perspective, that they are undertaken as efficiently as possible. However this should not be at the expense of placing undue burden upon users and carers in the completion of these documents.

Desirable technical features of standardized assessment schedules

In addition to the design elements, there are a number of technical criteria for assessment instruments.

How was the instrument developed?

It is important to know whether elderly people were included in the development of the instrument or whether it was developed by using volunteer USA college students? It is widely accepted that social support is an important factor in promoting the health of older people. However many of the available measures were developed by using students rather than older people. In studies developed with older people were people from particular groups (e.g. the very old, those of low social class or from minorities) included? Hence before adopting an instrument for inclusion in an assessment schedule the population for which it was developed must be closely scrutinized to see if it is transferable to the local setting.

The validity of the instrument

This describes the degree to which an instrument actually measures what it claims to measure. Users also need to consider if what is being measured is relevant to their context. For example the widely used Barthel index was not developed to measure 'disability' but rather to estimate patients needs for nursing care. Although this is a widely used measure, we do need to note that its original development may have been for an application rather different to its present use.

Many of the tools used in the assessment of older people, such as social support or disability, are subjective and there is no 'gold standard' with which to make comparisons as to the accuracy (or validity) of these tools. Consequently instruments are reviewed for content (or face) validity and their adherence to the principles of good questionnaire design. However, this approach is not without its problems. For example the words and phrases used in instruments may be culturally specific. The American version of the SF–36 asks if people feel 'lonesome and blue' and another asks if they are 'full of pep'. These are translated in the UK version as downhearted and low and full of life respectively. Similarly, the ISEL measure of social support includes the following satement 'if I needed a ride to the airport very early in the morning, I would have a hard time finding someone to take me'. The applicability of this question to a population of UK elders is probably very limited.

Sensitivity and specificity

Sensitivity and specificity relate to the ability of the instrument to identify true positives, that is people who have dementia or community care needs (known technically as sensitivity) and true negatives, that is people who are not depressed or who do not need help (technically termed specificity). These concepts are very important when screening for disease (e.g. breast cancer). However in many of the situations in which assessment instruments are used with older people these concepts are difficult to compute because of the difficulties involved in establishing an 'accurate' diagnosis. However, mental health, especially cognitive function, is recommended to form part of the complex assessment. In this case, it is the clinical examination which forms the 'gold standard' and it is against this that the performance of the instrument is judged. We can be certain that most assessment schedules used with older people vary in their sensitivity and specificity and therefore the degree to which the results identify 'real' needs. For example, the mini mental state examination (MMSE), a dementia screening tool, is known to have high false positive rates for poorly educated people and high false negative rates for well educated ones. This means that people from a poor educational background are more likely to be identified as having poor cognitive function when, in fact, they have no such impairment. Conversely, well educated people with impaired function are likely to be misclassified as well. Similarly many of our currently used cognitive function tools have been developed for use with white Anglo-Saxon populations and may not, therefore, be appropriate for use with older people from minority communities and may produce erroneously high (or low) prevalence rates.

Reliability

This describes the degree to which an instrument reproduces the same results under the same conditions. It is an important issue in the community care setting where assessments will be undertaken by a variety of different individuals and in a variety of different settings. Indeed, Leicester *et al.* (1996) report that, in an eight week trial period in Wandsworth, 43 different people were involved in undertaking community care assessments. We need to be confident that all those using the instrument do so correctly and that, if assessments are aggregated to inform population level developments, any differences seen between localities truly reflect differences in need and not differences between how the assessors use the instrument. We also need to be confident that elderly people assessed by different people receive equal treatment. Therefore, we must be convinced of the reliability of the schedule.

Availability of assessment schedules for elderly people

Given the requirements noted above it is, perhaps, not surprising that standard rigorously tested assessment instruments are available for only a limited number of the elements of the needs profile proposed by the DoH (RCP/BGS, 1992). However, as these instruments cover the social support/social network, disability, activities of daily living and mental health and carer aspects of the needs profile, such instruments are invaluable for the 'heart' of the assessment process. As we will see below most local authorities have designed their own schedules and it is not clear whether they have considered the issues covered already.

CONTENT OF ASSESSMENT SCHEDULES

To date there are only limited data on the nature and content of assessment schedules. Reviews by Leicester (1994) and Herrington (1996) reveal that most local authorities have opted for a structured type of assessment form. The findings of these studies may probably be generalized from the two study areas of the former South West Thames RHA and Greater London respectively. Such forms are characterized by a mixture of structured questions, answers and checklists. However most forms included space for the assessor (or the assessed) to make their own comments. These two studies identified only one borough which adopted a radically different approach. Here the assessment, apart from identifying the topics to be covered, was almost totally unstructured and it was left to the assessor to guide and structure the assessment. The structured and standardized approach to assessment means that there is a strong element of standardization across assessments and the questions asked/topics covered do not reflect the views or biases of the individual undertaking the assessment. However, it also means that the 'agenda' for the needs assessment is already set and it is not clear how older people can ensure that their needs are articulated within such a heaviliy prescribed and structured process. Here we have two opposing and contradictory pressures; the desire for standardization and the desire to enable the process to be 'needs led'.

Who does the assessment?

Assessment is clearly an important aspect of community care as it lays the foundation upon which the rest of the policy stands (or falls). Deciding on who should undertake assessments is, therefore, a very important aspect of the implementation of community care. Leicester and Pollock (1996) report that in the eight departments they studied assessments were being undertaken by a range of different staff including social workers, occupational therapists, administrative staff and other members of the departments. Over an eight week period in Wandsworth, Leicester *et al.* (1996) report that 43 different professionals were involved in the process of assessment. In that survey, social workers undertook 43% of the assessments and 34% were by occupational therapists. However when we consider only older people (which represents 66% of assessments) then 50% were undertaken by occupational therapists and 25% each by social workers and domiciliary assessors.

Furthermore, in some areas the assessment was done by the older person themselves through the completion of a self-completion document which was usually very long and which they returned to social services departments for them to take action (Herrington, 1996). Clearly, this an element of community care which is, again, being approached in a variety of different ways by the agencies involved.

What comprises assessments?

Table 4.8 Analysis of topics covered by complex assessment forms

Topic	Leicester and Pollock (1996) n = 8	Herrington (1996) n = 22
Client profile	8	22
Carer profile	6	22
Activities of daily living	8	22
Mobility	8	21
Mental health	8	22
Sensory function	8	17
Social support	8	19
Leisure	6	11
Risk assessment	4	7
Transport/access	6	6

We noted earlier that the DoH, and indeed other commentators had proposed a variety of different topic areas which should be included in a complex assessment of an older persons needs. Table 4.8 shows that most of the local authorities studied by Herrington (1996) and Leicester (1994) included measures of health status and activities of daily living. However other areas suggested by the DoH such as transport, carer needs and risk assessment were much less well recorded. Hence in the two areas studied there was a broad consensus on the areas included (and excluded) from a complex assessment of an older person's needs.

Despite a broad agreement about the basic topic areas covered, detailed examination of the questions included in these broad areas revealed enormous heterogeneity in how local authorities had operationalized these concepts. For example all of the local authorities reviewed by Herrington and Leicester recorded details of the clients mental health. Clearly this is a broad aspect of the ability of the older person to remain at home and includes cognitive function, depression/anxiety, short-term problems such as bereavement and possibly major psychotic disorders which the person may have had all their life. Herrington (1996) reports that, behind the apparent consensus about the need to measure mental health, there was an enormous variation in how the authorities she reviewed had actually gone about this. A minority of authorities had comprehensively attempted to review this aspect of people's lives by including all the aspects noted above and they had used standardized assessment schedules to record this. The vast majority had confined their attention to recording the cognitive function of the person being assessed. Furthermore, cognitive function was tackled in a variety of ways from the employment of a validated set of questions through to a note to the assessor to comment if the client 'appeared' to have impaired cognitive function. The usefulness of many of these assessment tools in identifying those who had impaired mental function is probably open to question.

Table 4.9 Use of standardized measures in complex assessments

	Leicester and Pollock (1996)	Herrington (1996)
Activities of daily living	4/8	8/22
Mobility	5/8	3/22
Mental health	4/8	0/22
Sensory impairment	5/8	2/17
Social support	2/8	1/19

There are a variety of standard measures available for some of the topic areas consistently included in the complex assessment forms used with older people. Table 4.9 reveals that, with the exception of the use of the Barthel scale to measure activities of daily living, most schedules did not include the use of standardized measures where they were available. It is interesting to speculate as to why these standardized measures were not used. It could be that the designers of the assessment forms were unaware of their existence or considered them inappropriate for use in this setting. Clearly, we need to look in more detail at the content of assessment forms and how the questions are asked. Also, to assess if the use of standardized measures would improve the effectiveness of the assessment process for older people.

There is one very glaring omission from the list of topics included in the assessment forms reviewed by both Herrington (1996) and Leicester (1996) and this is the consideration of the older person's identification of their own needs. In few of the schedules reviewed was there a space for this. This would seem to be in almost total opposition to the spirit of the community care changes which is supposed to be needs-led rather than service-led. The assessment schedules reviewed by these two authors appear to be less service-led in the types of questions asked. However, they are still making very profound assumptions about the factors which are important for maintaining older people at home and the aspects of independence which are important to them. For example, few forms bother to record details about many of the aspects relating to 'quality of life' while collecting considerable detail about people's ability to do household chores (but not other aspects like gardening or house maintenance). This echoes the work in the field of health outcome measures where there has been comparatively little interest in finding out what patients perceive as the benefits which they expect to result from treatment (Victor, 1996b).

Leading on from this is a point relating to the 'tone' of the assessments and the questions asked. Typically the questions asked take a 'problem-centred' approach. Hence the activities of daily living questions ask about the client's inability to perform various tasks such as washing, dressing and shopping. Such an approach focuses very much upon the 'weaknesses' of clients and not on their strengths or potential. It could be argued that it is equally important that assessment identifies the potential and strengths of clients which could be developed in order to promote independent living in the community.

PRACTITIONERS' ATTITUDES TOWARDS COMMUNITY CARE AND ASSESSMENT

The introduction of the community care changes has brought in its wake very fundamental changes in the function of social service departments and the staff that work within them. Caldock (1993) provides some insights into social workers' perceptions of these changes. The results of her interviews revealed a split in opinions about the merits of the system ranging from those who saw it as a recognition of the 'good practice' to which the social work profession had been striving and those who saw it solely in terms of a desire by central government to restrict funding and limit service provision.

The focus upon assessment of needs has involved a fundamental shift in the working practice of those who are employed in social service departments. Instead of simply identifying the types of services a person might need the emphasis is now upon identifying the full range of social care needs irrespective of the existence of services/resources to meet these needs. Caldock (1993) reports that her interviewees were very concerned about the effects, upon both assessor and client, of identifying needs which could not be met. A clear need for training and professional development in the field of assessment was articulated as this was such a radical change in the method of working. It is not clear how well this demand has been fulfilled.

There were other aspects of the changes which were sources of concern. Taking responsibility for holding a budget was felt to compromise the process of assessment, as this group of respondents saw themselves very clearly as acting as 'advocate' for the clients and their needs. The referral process, who should undertake assessments and the willingness (or otherwise) of different professional

groups/agencies to accept each other's assessments were all raised as issues caus-
ing concern. This small scale study in Wales highlighted many of the issues concerning the implementation of community care which still require resolution. In
particular the future of the social work profession and its role within community
care is under review. Will social workers spend all their time doing assessments
and providing care packages and not doing 'social work'? We need a longer
experience of the implementation of the legislative changes before we can defini-
tively answer many of these questions.

THE EXPERIENCE OF ASSESSMENT

In this section we will consider, using available data, how the assessment system
has been working in the first few years of its implementation. We will look at the
source and number of assessments being undertaken and the experiences of older
people and their carers of the new system. Hughes (1995) provides a comprehensive overview of the more detailed aspects of how practitioners should approach
the assessment of older people and some models of good practice for working with
older people.

For an assessment to be undertaken, older people (and indeed other client groups)
must make contact with the social services department. Do older people and their
carers know about the new system and how to use it? We have seen that part of a
local authority's new responsibilities are to make information about the system and
how to use it widely available. An early report from the Carers Association (Warner,
1994) indicated that 73% of carers (of any age dependent) knew about the changes
and 79% knew where to get help. However, the report notes that carers of people
aged 65 years and over (and who are likely to be elderly themselves – see Chapter
6) were less likely to know about the changes and where to get help. Although this
research was carried out immediately following the implementation of the changes
it is not clear if users and carers are much better informed now.

Despite the less than universal recognition of the community care legislation a
large percentage of referrals, between a third and a half, are generated by the informal sector (e.g. family, friends, carers or the person themselves) (Table 4.10).
Leicester (1994) reports that the majority of referrals (54%) come via a telephone
call.

Table 4.10 Source of referrals for community care assessment – all ages (%)[a]

	Leicester et al.	*LMGB*
Informal (carer, relative)	51	36
Hospital	15	24
Primary care	16	11
Other	18	29

[a]Derived from: Leicester *et al.*, 1996, Table 3.4; LGMB, 1996, Table 3

How many assessments are being undertaken? Leicester (1994) reported that in one London borough, Wandsworth, approximately 4000 assessments were being undertaken annually. The majority of assessments (74%) were for people aged 65 years and over. Over an eight week survey period, 234 assessments were undertaken by 10 teams working in Merton and 66% were for older people. Hence, the main group of people currently receiving assessments are older people and this is a pattern which is probably typical of the national picture.

Table 4.11 Community care assessment: 1st January–30th June 1996; per 1000 aged 65 years or over[a]

	Referrals	*Assessment*	*Percentage referrals assessed*
Counties	142.7	88.1	61.7
Metro-authorities	160.0	114.3	71.4
London	272.8	225.4	82.6
England	151.8	98.8	65.0

[a]Derived from: LGMB, 1996, Tables 12 and 13

Clearly the absolute number of assessments being undertaken by specific local authorities will vary because of their differing population sizes. Table 4.11 presents information about the number of referrals and assessments being undertaken by a sample of local authorities across the country. This shows that, nationally, about two-thirds of referrals appear to result in an assessment and that rates of both referral and assessment are highest in inner London and lowest in the counties. These data do not distinguish between the type of assessment (i.e. complex or simple). However, for the year 1993/94 approximately one-third of assessments included in a national survey were defined as complex (LGMB, 1994).

What areas of needs are being assessed? A survey in Merton looked at what needs were being assessed by different types of assessors for all the major client groups. Although the numbers were small, some interesting issues emerge from these data. First, regardless of profession, older people are most likely to be assessed for the 'classic' activities of daily living. Almost universally activities such as self-care were assessed (by over 85% of OT assessments, 82% of social worker assessments and 68% of domiciliary services assessments). Virtually no assessors looked at relationships, accommodation, community skills or racial/cultural/spiritual aspects of an older person's needs. Clearly the assessors were making assumptions about the 'unimportance' of these issues to the older people they saw. Second, there were differences between groups in some of the dimensions assessed. For example approximately two-thirds of social work assessments looked at protection of the older person from physical/mental abuse; aspects included in under 10% of assessments undertaken by other groups. Consequently the professional perspective of the person undertaking the assessment is clearly influencing the direction followed. This may mean that some important needs of older people may remain obscure.

What is the outcome of the assessment process? We will look in detail at the types of services received following assessment in a later part of the book (Chapters 5 and 7). Here we will confine our comments to the broad outcome of the assessment process. Leicester (1994) examined outcomes for 1103 assessments in Wandsworth. This revealed that 55% had services provided following the assessment, 10% had services discontinued, 24% were given no services and the remainder (11%) were referred elsewhere. This is in broad agreement with the review of a sample of local authorities nationally which revealed that 27% of assessments resulted in no services being provided (LGMB, 1996).

Did the outcome of the assessment vary with the needs of the person assessed? Table 4.12 shows that services were less likely to be provided/maintained to the highest categories of needs. Additionally, 29% of this group had services discontinued or were not given services. it is not clear as to why this is so high. It might reflect people dying or moving away but is clearly an area for research.

Table 4.12 Outcome of assessments (all ages) by need category: Wandsworth, October–December, 1993[a]

	Percentage outcome		
Outcome	High need	Moderate need	Low need
New service provided	30	36	23
Existing service changed	10	13	6
Addition to existing service	10	9	3
Unchanged services	10	8	10
No service provided	11	16	42
Referred to home area	11	10	10
Service discontinued	18	8	4
N	400	300	403

[a]Derived from: Leicester, 1994, Table 6

There are only very limited data available as to how users and carers perceive the assessment process. Warner (1994) reports on the experiences of a variety of carers. He reports that the majority of carers (70%) felt that the assessment had been thorough but that 40% were felt not to meet the needs of the person assessed and 51% did not meet the needs of the carer. Just over a half (51%) of carers felt that the assessment process was limited by financial considerations.

How did it feel to be assessed? Comments documented by Warner (1994, p. 27) give us some insight into the daunting and apparently bureaucratic nature of the experience. For example one carer stated '... She (social worker) left the (assessment) form with me. It was 16 pages long. She did not go over it with me'. Another said 'We were given one (assessment) we did not want', while another said 'Somebody from the home care services came along with reams and reams of paper and did an assessment of my wife ... The net result was that they could not offer us anything'. In our search to develop methodologically sound assessment schedules we must not forget the people who are experiencing what could easily become a rather intrusive and authoritarian experience.

CONCLUSION

In theory, at least, assessment should be a way of identifying the needs of older people (and indeed other client groups) which will enable them to remain living in the community. However this is a task, which we have illustrated, which is not without challenges. There are clearly problems in how the assessment is undertaken, who undertakes it and which issues are covered. Furthermore, the process needs to ensure that the information provided by the assessment process remains confidential. It is not yet clear how the assessment process is enabling users and carers the opportunity to take 'risks' and exercise real choice over options for their care.

There are some further issues which require consideration. There is a clear tension between assessment as a 'user- and needs-led' activity and the requirement to target services at those in greatest 'need'. Hence, on one level at least, assessment is a way of rationing services. Indeed the legislation is quite unambiguous that services are to be provided 'within existing means'. Hence Meredith (1995) has suggested that assessments are not reflecting individuals needs but only those which authorities feel they can meet.

In theory at least the assessment process could be a means of empowering users and carers. We might speculate that even if assessment identified needs which could not be met then users/carers could use these data to campaign for more/better/different services. More broadly such evidence about 'unmet' needs could be fed back into the planning process. However these might be unduly optimistic views upon the potential of the assessment process. A longer experience of the implementation of the assessment process will enable us to judge whether this optimism is well founded.

5

Care in the community: the role of the formal sector

INTRODUCTION

In this chapter we examine the contribution of formal community care services (excluding the long stay sector which is dealt with elsewhere) in maintaining older people in the community. We concentrate upon looking at the expenditure upon community care services, levels of service provision and examine the pattern of service utilization by older people. We will also consider how older people feel about the types and range of services provided for them. To what degree do services meet the 'real' needs identified by older people themselves?

Although most of this chapter concentrates on the provision of services that are responding to social care needs we also discuss health services, voluntary services, housing and income support agencies where appropriate. Of necessity much of the data presented relates to the period prior to and immediately following the implementation of the community care changes. However this will act as a 'benchmark' against which the changes may be evaluated. Furthermore, by providing data regarding service provision over a longer time frame we can more reliably examine trends in the provision of community care services.

HOW MUCH DO WE SPEND ON COMMUNITY CARE?

Given the large number of agencies potentially involved in the provision of community care, this is a difficult question to answer with any accuracy. According to estimates compiled by Robins and Wittenberg (1992) (Table 1.1), in England (1989–90) total public expenditure on health and social services for elderly people amounted to £11 350 million. This represents about half (47%) of the total public expenditure in these areas. *Per capita* expenditure increases markedly with age. There is an approximate five-fold increase in the amount spent per head for those aged 85 years and over (£3995 per annum) as compared with those aged 65–74

(£865 per head). Furthermore, this is an underestimate as it does not include expenditure on pensions or other important areas such as housing.

Laing (1993) has estimated the amount of NHS, and local authority expenditure per annum on community care services in the UK for the year from April 1992 (Table 5.1). These data are an underestimate because of the exclusion of the services provided by the former Family Health Services Authorities from the calculation (e.g. general practitioners, practice nurses, opticians, dentists, etc.). Overall, 82% of all NHS/local authority community care service expenditure is accounted for by older people. Older people are, as this table shows, the main consumer group for the services provided ranging from the provision of aids/adaptations, day care to the provision of district nursing services.

Table 5.1 Estimated expenditure on long-term care for people living in their own homes: UK, 1992[a]

| | Expenditure (£ million) | | |
	Total	Those aged 65+	% 65+
NHS			
district nursing	891	669	75
day-care	67	51	76
chiropody	79	71	90
Total NHS	1037	791	76
Local authority			
home care	815	701	86
social work	293	238	81
day-care	130	130	100
meals	90	90	100
other	85	85	100
aids and adaptations	74	42	57
User charges	124	107	86
Net local authority	1363	1179	87
Total public expenditure	2400	1970	82

[a]Derived from: Laing, 1993, Table 3

Laing (1993) estimates the annual expenditure on community care plus long-stay care at £7132 million per annum of which £6336 million (89%) is accounted for by older people. We will examine the issue of the funding of long-term nursing/residential care later (Chapter 7). This total represents about 1% of total GDP and is a figure which is quoted with alarm and consternation by politicians, civil servants and social commentators. However, to put these data into context, it is important to note here the contribution made by the 'informal sector'. This relates to the caring contribution made by family, friends and relatives which we consider in detail in Chapter 6. Laing (1993) estimates that, in one year, the 'value' of this care (costed at £7 an hour) was £39 100 million of which 83% (£32 500 million) was received by older people.

Table 5.1 presents an overview of the amount of money spent upon maintaining older people in the community. However it is the local authorities who have day-to-day responsibility for the financial aspects of community care as defined by the 1993 reforms. The funding of local government is a technical and complex issue outside the remit of this book, although we have touched upon some of the main issues (Chapter 2). We noted that a basic understanding of the funding system is important for understanding some of the debates now surrounding the implementation of community care at the local level. The Department of the Environment (DoE) using a set of 'needs criteria' allocates a block grant to each local authority. Although the money to be used for community care is not 'ring-fenced' within the overall allocation, the DoE do make assumptions, known as standard spending assessments (SSAs) as to what each local authority should be spending on their personal social services. Means and Smith (1995) consider the sums allocated are inadequate for meeting the community care objectives set by the Department of Health (DoH). They argue that, as a consequence of inadequate overall funding, local authorities are having to reduce their expenditure on community care to meet commitments elsewhere in their budget, reduce other services to fund community care or try to generate income by introducing (or increasing) charges for services. We will return to the issues of charging for services later in this chapter. However as Table 5.1 shows, 86% of money raised in user charges is derived from older people; hence older people as well as being major users of care are also major contributors.

Variations in community care expenditure: geographical aspects

We noted above that older people are significant users, in financial terms, of the overall community care budget of both health and local authorities. However, these data relate to the country as a whole. The next question to ask is how does expenditure on community care services vary locally. This is not easy to answer for individual health authorities. However local authorities do publish data about the percentage of their social service (community care) budget accounted for by different care groups. These data are slightly difficult to use because older people and those with physical handicaps are treated as a single group. Table 5.2 shows that in England (1993–94) 40% of all social services expenditure related to older people (and the physically handicapped). The percentage expenditure accounted for by older people was greatest among shire counties (42%) and lowest in London (32% inner London and 36% outer London). Similarly when we look at budgets (rather than expenditure) for residential/nursing care and day/domiciliary care a similar but slightly more complex pattern emerges (Table 5.3). Counties spend a higher percentage of their residential/nursing home budgets on older people than London boroughs but a much lower percentage on day/domiciliary care. This may reflect local preferences for services, different patterns of need or existing patterns of supply (or indeed some combination of these factors). To some degree the variations in expenditure reflect the percentage of older people in the population served. At a very crude level, therefore, expenditure relates to differing patterns of need as suggested by the population profile of these different types of areas.

Table 5.2 Social services expenditure (in percentage) on older or physically disabled people: England, 1993-94

	65+	85+	Living alone	Expenditure
Shire counties	16.8	1.8	32.0	42
Metro areas	16.6	1.6	35.5	40
Inner London	15.4	1.4	41.7	32
Outer London	14.7	1.7	34.1	36
England	15.7	1.7	33.4	40

Table 5.3 Community care budgets in England: 1995–96, percentage budget accounted for by older people[a]

	Percentage budget accounted for by older people		
	Residential/nursing home	Domiciliary	Total
Counties	72.2	54.8	65.4
Metro area	64.7	62.8	69.8
London	62.8	77.7	68.4
England	71.8	57.9	66.4

[a]Derived from: LGMB, 1996, Table 5

Variations in community care budgets

Allocation between types of services and providers

There were two clearly stated aims in the community care changes. First, to reduce the amount of money being spent on long-term care (especially that provided in private nursing and residential homes). Second, the changes were intended to develop the 'mixed economy' of provision by stimulating private sector providers in both the long-term and domiciliary sectors. Analysis of local authority budgets and expenditure can shed some light on how successful local authorities have been in achieving these objectives.

In 1994–95 residential/nursing care accounted for 59.3% of local authority community care budgets; this had increased to 61.5% for the year 1995–96 (Table 5.4). So, over this rather short time scale there was little obvious evidence of a downward trend in this type of expenditure. However the use of the private sector to provide services has increased over this period from 39.8% in 1994–95 to 49.3% in 1995–96. While each of the three types of administrative area shown in Table 5.4 have reported an increase in the percentage of the budget to be spent in the private sector, this trend is most enthusiastically demonstrated by the counties. This might reflect greater political enthusiasm for this policy change or the greater existing size of the private sector.

Table 5.4 Allocation of community care budgets in England 1994–1996[a]

	Percentage on residential/ nursing home		Percentage spent in independent sector	
	94/95[b]	95/96	94/95[b]	95/96
Counties	58.3 (54.7)	60.9	45.1 (40)	53.6
Metro areas	61.1 (69)	62.3	29.4 (36.5)	41.4
London	65.4 (65.5)	62.6	41.2 (39.5)	44.9
England	59.3 (59.2)	61.5	39.8 (39)	49.3

[a]Derived from: LGMB, 1996, Tables 1, 2 and 6
[b]Projected expenditure (1994–1995) with actual expenditure in parenthesis

The balance of expenditure between different types of local authority services for older people is shown in Table 5.5. Nationally, just over half (51%) of local authority expenditure for older people is accounted for by residential/nursing home care and almost one third (29%) by the home care services. However, as Table 5.5 shows, the balance of care varies across the country. Compared with the overall national picture and the shire counties, in London a lower percentage of expenditure is represented by the residential/nursing home sector and a greater percentage by the day care/home care services. From these data we cannot determine the reasons underpinning this variation in the balance of care. However, we may speculate that it reflects a differential supply of services, variation in the needs/preferences of clients or some combination of these factors.

Table 5.5 Percentage of gross social services expenditure for older and physically disabled clients spent in different areas: England, 1993–94[a]

	Percentage budget spent on				
	Residential	Day-care	Home help	Meals	Other
Shire counties	55	7	29	3	7
Metro areas	50	7	31	3	9
Inner London	45	9	29	7	10
Outer London	44	10	31	7	7
England	51	8	29	4	8

[a]Derived from: DoH, 1995b, Table E3

THE USE OF COMMUNITY CARE SERVICES: HEALTH CARE SERVICES

Although the focus of this book is upon community care for older people it is impossible to review this subject without reference to the health care sector. We have already seen that, conceptually, there is a problem in defining the boundary between health care and social care. More fundamentally, the policy of community based care would founder if it were not underpinned by a comprehensive medical service. In this section, we examine the use made by older people of both the primary and secondary health care sectors.

Primary health care is perhaps one of the key services for achieving the objective of community care; the maintenance of elderly people in their own homes for as long as possible. The GP, by annual health checks for all those aged 75 years or more on their list, has a key role in the surveillance and monitoring of older people and in determining unmet needs for care. Regrettably, however, the failure to institute a standardized method of conducting these assessments means that much of the data collected are of little value in either identifying older people 'at risk' or in developing population based needs assessment. Additionally, the GPs are important because of their 'gatekeeper' function whereby they can control the entry of older people into the care system by referrals to appropriate agencies. They are also important in making referrals to hospital and community based services.

What use do older people make of the primary care team? This is slightly difficult to answer as data are not routinely collected about consultations between older people and all the different members of the primary care team. However, data are available for three principle members of the team; the GP, the practice nurse and the community nurse. Each of these is now considered in turn.

Consultations with GPs

Annually, it is estimated that approximately 75% of those aged 65 years and over will visit their family doctor (Victor,1991). According to the GHS, 47% of those aged 65 years and over consulted their GP at the surgery and 11% had a home visit in the three months before interview (Table 5.6). One important dimension of the utilization of the family doctor's service by older people is the location of the consultation. For those aged 65–69 years, 6% had a home visit as did 31% of those people aged 85 years or over. At all ages, women are more likely to have a home consultation than their male contemporaries. Older people are much more likely than any other group within the population to see their GP at home. Forward projection of current trends implies a potential increase in demand for home consultations.

How have consultations rates with GPs changed over time? The most complete data about time trends in GP consultations is available from the GHS. This provides data on the percentage of people consulting a GP in the last 14 days for the period 1972 to 1994 (Table 5.7). The percentage of older people consulting their GP in the 14 days before interview shows some evidence of increased utilization rates, especially for the 65–74 age group (rather than those aged 75 years or over). A similar pattern is observed for the average number of consultations. These data show only limited evidence of increased demand for GP services from older people over the past two decades. However, if future generations of elders show the same patterns of service use, then GP services will experience increased demands for their services simply because of the demographic changes noted in Chapter 3.

Table 5.6 Consultation with GPs in the three months prior to interview (%): Great Britain, 1994[a]

	Age										
	65–69		70–74		75–79		80–84		85+		All/65+
	M	F	M	F	M	F	M	F	M	F	M	F
GP at surgery	49	47	49	49	54	49	51	42	48	33	50	46
GP at home	4	6	8	8	8	14	16	21	18	35	8	13
Nurse at surgery	15	17	15	16	23	21	15	18	17	14	17	17

[a]Derived from: GHS, 1996, Table 6.43

Table 5.7 Trends in GP consultation for those aged 65 years and over, 1972–1994[a]

	Percentage consulting a GP in previous 14 days				Average number of consultations per person per year			
	65–74		75+		65–74		75+	
	M	F	M	F	M	F	M	F
1972	12	15	19	20	4	5	7	7
1979	14	17	16	23	5	5	5	8
1981	13	16	17	20	4	5	6	6
1983	18	18	20	21	5	6	7	7
1985	15	17	19	20	5	5	6	7
1987	17	18	22	22	6	6	7	7
1989	16	19	19	22	5	6	6	7
1991	17	19	21	19	5	6	7	6
1992	18	21	22	21	6	6	7	6
1993	21	20	22	23	6	6	7	7

[a]Derived from: GHS, 1995, Tables 6.9 and 6.10

Consultations with practice nurses

Older people are also extensive users of the practice nursing service (Table 5.6). In a three month reference period, 17% of those aged 65 years have seen a practice nurse. Practice nurses appear to be most heavily involved with those in the 75–79 years age range. This might reflect their role in carrying out the over 75 years assessments and the possibly more complex nature of the care required by those aged over 80 years (or the reduced mobility of this group rendering practice based consultation impossible).

Community nursing services

District nursing and, to a lesser degree, health visiting services are important for older people as part of the framework of primary health care services. Overall about half (47%) of the visits undertaken by district nurses were to those aged 65 years and over compared with 10% of health visitor contacts (Victor, 1991). As noted earlier over 80% of the district nursing budget was accounted for by work with those aged 65 years and over.

Data provided by the 1994 GHS do not distinguish between district nurses/health visitors. In 1994, approximately 6% of those aged 65 years and over were in receipt of district nursing/health visiting services (Table 5.8). So, although older people form the main client group for the community nursing service and account for the majority of the budget, the service actually only covers a small minority of the elderly population. This remains true even though utilization rates increase significantly with age. For example 2% of those aged 65–69 years are in receipt of district nursing/health visitor care compared with about 15% of those aged 85 years and over.

Table 5.8 Contact with district nurse/health visitor in previous month (%): Great Britain, 1994[a]

	M	F	All
65–69	1	3	2
70–74	3	4	3
75–79	4	7	6
80–84	9	14	12
85+	18	19	19
All 65+	4	7	6

[a]Derived from: GHS, 1996, Table 6.46

Services are provided for only a minority of those in greatest need. Of those who need help with walking outdoors – 23% receive district nursing visits as do 16% of those who need help getting out of bed and 17% of those who need help showering and 15% of those who need help dressing (GHS,1996). Of those who live alone and need help getting outdoors, getting up steps or with bathing less than one fifth receive visits from the district nurse (11%, 15% and 12% respectively) (Table 5.9).

Barrett and Hudson (1997) studied the workload of district nurses in a specific locality of London. Since the introduction of community care they report that nurses are caring for an older, frailer population and are undertaking more 'technical' nursing activities. What, they wonder, has happened to those less frail patients who had previously received district nursing (perhaps for bathing etc.). It is a feature of the debate about the community care changes; services are being targeted at those in greatest need but what about less intense 'preventative' work. This is an important point which needs to be borne in mind. It might be cost-effective to spend limited resources on those for whom there is some hope of preventing/delaying deterioration rather than the already very frail.

Table 5.9 Contact with district nurse/health visitor in previous month by household (%): Great Britain, 1994[a]

	Lives alone		Lives with spouse		Other	
	M	F	M	F	M	F
65–74	3	6	2	1	1	2
75+	12	13	7	10	7	11
All	5	13	3	4	2	6

[a]Derived from: GHS, 1996, Table 6.47

The role of health visitors with older people remains unresolved. Research has suggested that health visitors have a major role to play in screening and assessing the elderly (Vetter *et al.*, 1984). These activities are at the heart of community care. Health visitors are seen by their fellow health professionals as the group most suited to undertake this activity (Tremellen and Jones, 1989). The same study revealed that at least half the health visitors surveyed saw the focus of their work being on the pre-school child (0–5) age group which probably reflects the balance of their training where the emphasis is upon pre-school aged children. However, given the proven effectiveness of health visitors working with older people it might be appropriate to strengthen their training in this area.

The secondary care sector

Hospitals play a vital role in the provision of medical care for all members of the community but especially for older people. It is, for this group, the service which perhaps they use most extensively. Older people are the main consumer group catered for by the NHS. In 1990–91 45.5% of acute beds were occupied by those aged 65 years and more (Tinker *et al.*, 1994). The high utilization of hospital services by older people is further emphasized by looking at hospital admissions data (Table 5.10). Overall people aged 65 years and over accounted for 27.9% of all NHS admissions in England (29.2% of ordinary admissions and 22.6% of day cases) and 49% of total bed days. Both average and median duration of stay in hospital increase with age so that it is those people aged 85 years and over who have the longest average (35.6 days) and median (10 days) length of stay. Total hospital cases and ordinary admissions (in-patient cases) per 1000 population are three times higher for those aged 85 years and over as compared with those aged 65–74 years. However, the utilization of day case surgery peaks with the 75–84 years age group and then declines.

Table 5.10 Hospital utilization by age: England, 1990–91[a]

	65–74	75–84	85+
Hospital admissions per 1000	224.1	433.0	766.7
Day-cases per 1000	48.0	51.7	40.7
Total cases per 1000	272.1	487.1	807.3
Ordinary admissions (%)	12.2	12.2	4.8
Day-cases (%)	13.1	7.3	1.2
Total cases (%)	12.3	11.4	4.2
Bed days (%)	16.5	20.2	12.3
Mean stay (days)	19.0	23.3	35.6
Median stay (days)	5	7	10

[a]Derived from: DoH, 1994, Table 9

The above data relate to admission not to individual patients as one person may have multiple admissions to hospital. For data about the percentage of older people being admitted as in-patients or day patients we must use data from the GHS. This will be an under-estimate of the total percentage of older people being admitted to hospital as the sample excludes those living in nursing or residential homes. Given this caveat, in 1993, 9% of the population were admitted as in-patients to hospital compared to 11% of those aged 65 years and over (OPCS, 1995a). The percentage of the population reporting a hospital in-patient stay increases with age from 12% of those aged 65–74 years to 18% of those aged 75 years and over (Table 5.11). For the older age groups men have a higher rate of hospital admission than women. For those aged 75 years and over, 21% of men and 16% of women reported an in-patient stay in hospital in the previous year. This has remained fairly constant for the 65–74 years age group over the last 20 years, but has increased by 50% for males aged 75 years and over (15% in 1972 – 21% in 1993) and 33% for women (12% in 1972 to 16% in 1993) (Table 5.11). The average number of nights spent in hospital as an in-patient for those aged 65–74 years in 1993 was 13 days and 14 days for those aged 75 years and over (OPCS, 1995a). For the population as a whole in 1993, 5% attended hospital as a day patient in the previous year compared with 5% of those aged 65–74 years and 4% for those aged 75 years and over.

However, over the last decade there have been a significant reduction of 27.6% in the number of available acute hospital beds in England (Tinker *et al.*, 1994). Over the same period there has been a massive increase in throughput of patients treated. Tinker *et al.* (1994) report that between 1981 and 1991 the number of patients treated per bed increased by two-thirds. Hospital admission rates for older people appear to have increased markedly over the last decade (even allowing for changes in the method of data collection). This increase appears to have been most marked among those aged 75 years and over (Table 5.12). For example admission rates for those aged over 75 years appear to have doubled over the last 12 years. It is not clear what has brought about this change, but it is probably partly a reflection of a changed method of data collection. However, part of the increase is undoubtedly real. This may reflect a number of factors including an increased willingness to treat older people, a changed threshold for admission to hospital or the influence of repeated admission to hospital resulting from decreased length of stay.

Table 5.11 Trends in in-patient stays – population aged 65 years and over (%): Great Britain, 1982–93[a]

Year	Age			
	65–74		75+	
	M	F	M	F
1982	12	8	14	12
1985	13	18	17	13
1987	12	11	20	14
1989	12	11	17	17
1991	13	11	20	16
1992	16	11	18	17
1993	14	10	21	16

[a]Derived from: GHS, 1995, Table 6.21

Table 5.12 Hospital admission/discharge rates: England, 1979–1990/91

	Rate per 1000		
	65–74	75–84	85+
1979	145.6	216.1	325.0
1985	177.6	277.8	400.2
1990/91	272.1	487.1	807.3
Change (%)	86	225	248

This increased utilization of health services by older people has been achieved by significant reductions in the length of time people spend as in-patients and by the growth of day case treatment. However, the average length of stay in hospital for older people is usually longer than that for a young person with a similar medical condition. This reflects the multiple pathology which is often a feature of older people presenting with specific medical conditions. Very aggressive in-patient treatment regimens may result in 'sicker' patients being discharged back to the community with the resultant increased strain upon community care services.

The other elements of the secondary care sector are the out-patient and accident and emergency departments. Older people are also significant users of these types of services. In a three month reference period approximately one-fifth of older people visited either (or both) of these services (Table 5.13). Again there has been some increase in utilization rates over time with rates approximately doubling over the 20 years 1972–1993 (Table 5.13). This increase is observable for both men and women but is less marked for the general population (from 10% in 1972 to 14% in 1993).

Table 5.13 Use of A and E departments/outpatients: Population aged 65 years and over (%): Great Britain, 1972–1993[a]

	65–74		75+	
	M	F	M	F
1972	10	12	10	13
1975	11	12	12	10
1979	15	16	13	16
1981	14	16	14	16
1983	15	19	19	16
1985	15	18	19	17
1987	17	17	21	18
1989	18	19	16	19
1991	18	18	22	18
1992	20	22	21	22
1993	20	18	24	18

[a]Derived from: GHS, 1985, Table 6.18

Discharge from hospital back to the community

For many patients, irrespective of age, admission to an acute hospital constitutes only one phase of their medical career. Many patients need continuing care, follow-up or rehabilitation. A constant research theme into the hospital care of older people is the discharge from hospital back to the community. Discharge is, perhaps, the wrong term to use. This implies a severing of relationships when many will need continuing care; perhaps the term 'transfer' is a more accurate representation of the concept involved.

Consistently, research has demonstrated that the transfer of older clients from hospital back to the community can be very problematic. Older people more often sent home without adequate arrangements having been made for their continuing medical and community care (Marks, 1994). Some medical specialties, especially geriatric medicine, are much better than others at arranging effective transfer. This problem centres upon effective communication between hospital, community and local authority services. It remains unclear as to how the new community care changes will expedite or hinder such communications. However it is still the case that some older people remain in hospital for longer than is necessary because of the difficulties in organizing and providing appropriate community care services.

Issues in the provision of hospital care to older people

Delayed discharge and the 'inappropriate' use of acute beds

The most appropriate way of providing health care for older people within the hospital sector remains a point of contention. Should older people be treated by a specialist in age related geriatric medicine, or should they be cared for within mainstream services and specialties, or by specialists in the medicine of old age working within other specialisms?

There are protagonists for all these differing models of service provision. However the absence of any rigorous evaluative work makes it difficult to come to a scientific judgement about which is the best model of care to provide health care for older people. However, even if an age related service is established for those older people with acute medical problems, it seems likely that older people will remain high consumers of services provided in surgery and other specialist areas of modern medicine. As such all health care workers need to be aware of the particular issues relating to the appropriate care and management of older people, especially the organization of appropriate post-discharge care.

Alongside the debates about the most appropriate method of caring for the older patient are concerns about the 'blocking' of acute beds by older people who no longer need the facilities provided by an acute setting but who, for other reasons, cannot be discharged. Such patients are inevitably given the highly pejorative label 'bed blockers' which implies that it is the older person's fault that they cannot be discharged. This is highly inaccurate as it is almost always the case that people cannot be discharged because we cannot supply the appropriate services for them. People who fall into this category are at the interface of the health and social care systems and often experience prolonged stays in hospital because of the difficulties the two systems experience in organizing 'seamless' care across this administrative divide.

It has been stated that 'where patients have been assessed as not requiring continuing in-patient care ... they do not have a right to indefinitely occupy an NHS bed' (DoH, 1995). It is therefore very easy to assume that the issue of 'bed blocking' is new and has arisen because of the very recent changes in the health and social care systems. Under the current system social service departments are responsible for assessing and meeting care needs of people once they have been discharged. Such assessments have clearly to take place prior to discharge. This has led to a concern about the number of NHS beds 'blocked' by those either awaiting assessment or the provision of post-discharge care. According to the NHS Executive 6000 beds were 'blocked' (reported in the *Guardian*, 29/2/96) by those clinically fit for discharge but awaiting social services.

However, the issue of 'bed blocking' pre-dates the introduction of the 1991 NHS and Community Care changes. As early as 1948 the British Medical Association (BMA) commented 'unless sufficient residential homes are provided for old people ... hospital beds will inevitably become 'blocked' and the whole service will break down (Means and Smith, 1985, p. 175). Hence, almost since the creation of the post war welfare state there has been a concern that the hospital social care interface could, very easily for older people, become a 'bottleneck' which would bring down the whole system if not managed effectively. Consequently, there have been a number of studies which have sought to define methods of empirically identifying 'inappropriate' patients. They have sought to describe their characteristics and the reasons why such patients could not be discharged with the presumed aim of improving services so that such problems could be avoided. These studies have varied in the methodologies employed to under-take this type of research and the populations studied (Victor *et al.*, 1993). Consequently, this makes comparison across studies problematic and makes it difficult to assess if the introduction of community care has made things worse (or better).

Research in inner London reported that, in a cross sectional study, 19% of older patients (i.e. those aged 65 years and more) were defined by medical and/or nursing staff as 'bed blockers'. This estimate suggested that, overall, approximately 8% of acute beds were being 'blocked' by these patients (Victor *et al.*, 1993). However inappropriate bed use is not specific to older patients. Victor *et al.* (1993) report that only half of all patients identified as inappropriate were aged 65 years and more.

Why are patients described as being inappropriately placed? Victor (1990) reports that, from a study in inner London, the single most important reason cited was the need for nursing/institutional care (81%). Comparatively few elderly people were remaining in hospital because of problems in providing community based services. Although London appears to have the biggest problem with the supply of long-stay care, it is also an important issue throughout the rest of the country. Those older patients identified as being inappropriately placed within an acute unit almost always had a very real need for care. Indeed their health characteristics highlight the types of problems which often occupy the interface between acute and community care. Typically, patients identified as 'inappropriate', present problems such as incontinence, immobility, problems with self-care and dementia. These are likely to present considerable nursing care problems but they do not necessarily require continued in-patient care of the type provided by an acute unit (Victor, 1990).

This serves to highlight, yet again, one of the most persistent problems which has dogged the British welfare state since its creation; the boundary between health and social care. The architects of the original welfare state and the recent community care reforms made an assumption that it is easy to distinguish between these two different types of needs and therefore formulated services accordingly. As we have seen, for older people the distinction is not clear cut and, as they represent the largest single group using these welfare services, problems of definition, demarcation and definition abound. Means and Smith (1985, p. 183) quote Majorie Warren, an eminent pioneering geriatrician in 1951, as stating '... the elderly frequently fall between the two bodies – the individual not being sick enough to justify admission to hospital and yet too disabled for a vacancy in a (residential) home'. In a similar vein they quote an MP as identifying older people as falling in the 'no mans land ' between the NHS and local authority because '... they are not sick enough for hospital yet need more care and attention than can be given to them in their own homes ....' (Means and Smith, 1985, p. 183).

CARE IN THE COMMUNITY: LOCAL AUTHORITY SERVICES

Despite the moves towards local authorities being organizers, enablers and facilitators of care they still remain significant providers of care. The key services provided by local authorities include home care (home help) services, day-care, social work, meals services, occupational therapy and home aids/adaptations. Only very limited data are available which describe the provision and utilization of such services by older people. Three areas where data are available are home care, meals services and day-care. Each of these is now considered in turn.

The provision of home care services

In 1994, data from a one week survey conducted in England reported that local authorities provided/purchased 2 214 400 hours of home care/home help services for 537 600 households (DoH, 1995b). The number of hours of care provided increased by 31% between 1992 and 1994 and the number of households receiving such care by 1.7%.

Who provides home care purchased by the local authority? In 1994 the majority of contact hours (80.79%) and households (478 400 – 88.9%) received direct local authority provision. However the contribution made by private sector home care provision has increased significantly between 1992 and 1994. In 1994 it provided 19.1% of contracted hours and was used by 16.2% of households receiving home care; compared with 1.9% and 1.6% respectively in 1992. This reflects a large absolute increase in the contributions made from the private sector (32 300 contact hours and 8600 households in 1992 and 364 700 hours and 463 000 households in 1994) in response to direct government direction to increase the role of private sector providers.

Routine data such as that collected by the Department of Health give only very modest details about the extent of services provided. By simply dividing total hours of care provided by the number of households, we can estimate the average (mean) amount of service being provided. In 1992 an average of three hours service a week was provided to users; in 1994 the average was four hours. According to the DoH (1995b), the percentage of clients receiving an intensive service (over five hours per week) was 15% for direct local authority provision; 11% for the voluntary sector providers and 27% for those receiving private services. There appears to have been an increase in the percentage of users receiving an intensive service as in 1992 these percentages were 10, 3 and 9 respectively. However, if we exclude the 'intense' service users from the calculation of the amount of services received then these are reduced. Consequently most users of the home care service appear to receive a very minimal amount of service.

Provision of home meals

In England, during the sample survey week in 1994, 647 900 meals were 'purchased' by local authorities and were served to 209 300 people (this excludes meals served at lunch clubs/day centres). In 1994, 4% of meals were served and 7% of recipients had meals from private sector contractors (the comparable figures for direct local authority provision were 59% and 55.7%). It is in the provision of home meals that the voluntary sector is a major provider of services, serving 31% of meals provided (and 36.3% of recipients) (DoH,1995b). There has been some expansion of the home meals service. During the period 1992–1994 there was a 3% increase in meals delivered to people's homes and a 5% increase in people receiving meals at home.

Again, there are virtually no routine data as to the level of services received. One indicator of the intensity of the service being provided is provision of meals at the weekend. In 1992, 6% of meals were provided at the weekend compared with 7% in 1994. Hence, for most people this appears to be a service which is not provided on an intensive basis.

Provision of day care

The final element of community based forms of provision, for which data are made available routinely, is day-care places. Until 1991, official statistics reported the number of premises and day-care places available for the main client group. As of March 31st 1991 there were 750 premises in England providing 25 920 day-care places for elderly people (DoH, 1995b). However, current routine statistics do not distinguish between different client groups but do distinguish between providers. This reveals that, of the 3630 premises offering day-care, 63% were provided by the local authority and 33% by the voluntary sector. Similarly, of the 562 100 total places available 86% were provided by the local authority and 13% by the voluntary sector. Clearly in this aspect of community care the local authority has yet to make an impact.

Taking these three services together it is not obvious how much service is being received by individual clients and whether the level of service being provided can, in any way, 'prevent' those on the fringes of entry into long-term care from entering such accommodation.

Utilization of local authority provided/organized services

Having described the extent of provision available, how many of the population of older people are actually using these services? The GHS collects information about three local authority services: social worker contacts, home helps and home meals. Information is also collected about privately employed home help services (Table 5.14). Again, it is evident that local authority services are received by only a minority of older people and, overall, there is little gender difference in levels of receipt of these services. One interesting feature of this table is the use of privately employed home helps by older people. Overall, 7% of those aged 65 years and over employ a private home help compared with 8% receiving a local authority arranged home care service. We might speculate that this use of private home helps reflects an 'unmet need' for help with house care which is not being accepted by the local authority (perhaps because of their targeting and eligibility criteria). Wilson (1994) describes how, in a small sample of the over 75s living in London almost one half (41%) were paying for help with household cleaning. She suggest that the fairly widespread use of privately funded and arranged home care resulted from the interaction between both negative and positive forces. The negative forces were the well known deficiencies in state services (e.g. home helps not cleaning windows). More positively, Wilson speculates that privately arranged care was a way of maintaining autonomy and self-respect because it was initiated and controlled by the older people in a way in which state services could not be.

Table 5.14 Use of selected health and social care services by those aged 65 years and over (%): Great Britain, 1994[a]

	65–69		70–74		75–79		80–84		85+		All 65+	
	M	F	M	F	M	F	M	F	M	F	M	F
In last month												
home help (local authority)	2	3	2	5	7	10	9	18	25	27	5	10
home help (private)	3	4	3	5	8	11	9	11	14	17	5	8
meals on wheels	0	0	1	2	2	2	6	5	15	11	2	3
lunch club	1	2	1	2	3	4	6	8	7	7	2	4
day centre	2	2	2	3	4	4	5	7	6	5	3	4

Derived from: GHS, 1996, Table 6.46

One rationale underpinning the community changes has been the idea of 'better targeting' of services towards those 'most in need'. Do social care services show any evidence of being targeted at this group and has this targeting increased with the implementation of community care? One obvious group to target for services are the 'very old' (i.e. those aged 85 years and over).

Although levels of service use increase with age, services are still being received by a minority; 9% receive meals, 29% receive a home help and 7% have seen a social worker. Similarly, receipt of services by those living alone is also very limited. Services are also received by only a minority of those who experience difficulty with domestic tasks (Table 5.15) or cooking a meal (Table 5.16). Even for those who need help to cook a meal and who live alone, less than two thirds (60%) receive a local authority home help and just over one third (38%) are receiving home meals.

The now explicit aim of social service allocation is the targeting of services at the most frail and vulnerable. One group who would readily fall into this category are the very old. Consequently, we might expect that, with the introduction of community care, a large percentage of those aged 80 years and over would be receiving services. In 1980, 15% of men aged 80 years and over received a home help and 9% home meals (for women the percentages were 30 and 9 respectively) (Victor, 1987). Data for 1994 reveals virtually no change in the percentages of this age group receiving services. Home help was received by 14% of men and 22% of women, and meals by 9% of men and 8% of women. This does not provide any evidence to support the idea that services are being increasingly focused upon the most vulnerable.

Table 5.15 Receipt of services by those aged 65 years and over needing help with domestic tasks: Great Britain, 1994[a]

| | Percentage of those needing help with task | |
Task	Receiving LA home help	Receiving private home help
Washing and drying dishes	25	10
Vacuum floors	29	18
Clean windows inside	26	14
Hand washing	24	10
Household shopping	26	12

[a]Derived from: GHS, 1996, Table 6.50

Table 5.16 Receipt of services by those aged 65 years and over with difficulties cooking a meal: Great Britain, 1994[a]

| Provision of services to those needing help to cook a main meal | | |
Percentage receiving	All	Living alone
LA home help	31	60
Receiving meals	16	38
Visiting a lunch club	4	7
Visiting day centre	14	20

[a]Derived from: GHS, 1996, Tables 6.51 and 6.54

Developing packages of care

The analysis presented above has been an essentially singular one. Routine data, while presenting information about the use of individual services, is not a very good source of information about combinations of service use (or to use the jargon phrase packages of care). Given that the rationale of the community care changes is towards the development of care packages what information is available about the development of such entities.

Allen *et al.* (1992b) reviewed the care being received by 100 older people using social services and who were perceived as being on the 'fringes' of entry into residential care. They report that among their sample a care package, which implies multiple tailored services, was something of a euphemism. The majority of their sample (70%) had a care package provided of one or two services only for perhaps one or two days per week. They conclude that it was informal rather than formal care provision that prevented their sample from entering care. Similarly Bowling *et al.* (1993) confirm that large multiple service packages of care, as indicated by the receipt of four or more different services, remain the exception. However we need greater experience of the implementation of community care before we can judge whether older people really do receive worthwhile care packages or if this term is to retain its euphemistic nature.

User views on services

What do older people know about the services that are available and what do they think of the services they receive. Fell and Foster (1994) report that, among older people in Scotland, there was generally a high level of awareness of services such as district nursing, home helps and mobile meals services. Over 70% of all those interviewed were aware of these traditional community services. In this survey GPs (mentioned by 29%) and social work departments (mentioned by 22%) were the most important sources of information about services. However one third of respondents were unable to identify a specific source of information about such services. Clearly social service departments face a considerable challenge in providing information about the new system.

An important element of the new system is the emphasis upon ensuring the 'quality' of services provided, ensuring that users are happy with the services received and establishing appropriate procedures for monitoring service quality and complaints. Obtaining the views of users about the services they receive is problematic, especially where older people are concerned. Consistently surveys of older service users reveal very high levels of satisfaction when people are asked a direct question such as 'are you satisfied/dissatisfied with ... or how would you rate service x on a five point scale from very satisfied to very dissatisfied?'. However, by asking about the good/bad aspects of specific services, such as home helps, one can start to tease out the major sources of dissatisfaction (in this case staff turnover, perceived 'unreliability' of staff and the restricted nature of what they could/could not do) (Allen *et al.*, 1992b). Hence, if social service departments are to take seriously the task of eliciting user/carers views they will have to develop considerably more sophisticated methodologies than highly structured pre-coded self-completion questionnaires.

Who pays for social care services?

As noted earlier, a feature of the social care system, since its inception, has been the idea that users should be expected to contribute towards the care received. Charging for services has been adopted with varying degrees of enthusiasm by different local authorities. However with social care budgets under increased pressure it is likely that charging for services is going to become more important as local authorities seek to generate additional income. In 1991/92 almost all local authorities charged for meals, at least 80% charged for respite care and over two thirds charged for home care/day-care (Warner, 1994). It is likely that the percentage of authorities charging for services will increase and that users will be asked to pay a realistic cost as opposed to a more nominal (or flat rate) charge. Indeed, as local authority charges increase, we may see users and carers making increasing use of 'private' care arrangements as these may be cheaper and perceived as more flexible than formal local authority brokered arrangements.

According to Laing (1993), in 1992 78% of care provided to people in their own homes was publicly funded and supplied; 1% was publicly funded but supplied by the independent sector; 4% was publicly supplied but individually funded and 17% was independently provided and funded by individuals. Hence a significant percentage of older people are organizing and funding their own care (Wilson 1994).

Changes in service use: 1961 – 1991

In absolute terms the number of many local authority and community based health service staff and services have increased substantially over the past three decades (Tinker *et al.*, 1994). However these increases have barely kept pace with demographic changes. Table 5.17 shows that, despite variations in the way that data were collected, the percentage of those aged 65 years and over receiving some of the key community care services, such as home helps and home meals, have remained remarkably constant. The only significant change in the last five years has been the increased use of private home help services. While the percentage of the population aged 65 years and over receiving community nursing doubled between 1972 and 1985, the situation for health visiting remained constant.

Table 5.17 Use of services by those aged 65 years and over (%) in month prior to interview, 1965–1994[a]

	1962	1972	1976	1980	1985	1991	1994
Home help (LA)	5	5	8	9	7	9	8
Home help (private)	–	–	–	–	–	4	7
Meals on wheels	1	1	2	2	2	2	3
District nurse	2	5	5	5	5[b]	6[b]	6[b]
Health visitor	2	2	2	–	–	–	

[a]Derived from: Victor, 1991, Table 13.1; Goddard and Savage, 1994, Table 64; GHS, 1996, Table 6.45
[b]Includes health visitor

Changing patterns of service use with age

Much of the available research looking at the provision of care to older people is cross-sectional in nature. This means that we are collecting information at a single point. Clearly this approach is limited in that it tells us nothing about how service providers respond to people's changing needs as they grow older. To capture this information we need to take a longitudinal perspective following up people over time. Bowling *et al.* (1993) followed a sample of those aged 85 years and over (at baseline) over a two and a half year period and looked at changing patterns of service use. Deteriorating functional ability and living alone were the two factors which were related to increased service use over the follow-up period.

Use of services by minority elders

As has been noted previously one of the key changes which will take place in the composition of the elderly population in the next few years is the 'ageing' of the minority communities. As with other aspects of the study of ageing, it is important to remember that what is often referred to as 'the minority community' in fact covers a heterogenous collection of different groups. As Norman (1985) points out little is known about either the health status of elderly minority community members or their use of services. Fennel *et al.* (1988) comment upon the excess levels of particular conditions such as hypertension and stroke among older people from the Caribbean, and elevated ischaemic heart disease morbidity among elderly Asians. These authors comment upon the low levels of use of community based services by both elderly Asians and elderly Caribbeans. This contrasts with the situation for health services where Blakemore and Boneham (1994) observed that elderly Asians and Caribbean people used GP services more than white elders.

ALLOCATING CARE: WHO GETS HOME CARE?

As with entry to long-term care, local authorities use eligibility criteria to determine who does (and who does not) get domiciliary care to help maintain them in the community. A useful insight into the differential way eligibility criteria operate is from a survey undertaken by the ACC/AMA (1995). They attempted to compare eligibility criteria between 108 local authorities, of whom 74 (68%) replied but noted that 'it would have been very difficult to compare eligibility criteria from the documentation we received' (ACC/AMA, 1995). The study used 10 case studies (drawn from real examples) and asked responding local authorities if the individual would qualify for care, what type of care would be provided (nursing home, residential home, or home care) and then details about payment and amount of service. The case profiles were designed to present different types of need. In this section we deal with the four profiles relating to home care services and these are summarized in Table 5.18 as is the 'actual' outcome for each case.

Overall, the majority of local authorities surveyed reported that the cases described fell within their eligibility criteria. There is considerable consistency between types of authorities as to the 'theoretical' eligibility of these different types of need (Table 5.19). However there is some evidence that shire counties are less likely than urban authorities to accept these types of needs as falling within their eligibility criteria.

Of the needs described by the four case profiles, the majority were thought to be best met by home care services (Table 5.20). The amount of home care which was allocated to these hypothetical cases was largely very minimal. As Table 5.20 shows, only one case, the frail 84-year-old living alone, was likely to receive a significant allocation of home care. For the other three cases the majority of local authorities surveyed would have allocated under two hours of care a week. Two of the case profiles relate to elderly people newly discharged from hospital, one after an in-patient stay following a fall (case 2) and one after day case surgery following a cataract operation. In both these cases elderly people would, in previous times, have stayed in hospital for considerably longer than the current practice. This is an example of where responsibility for after care is being transferred from the health care sector to the social care sector. However such clients appear to have a low priority for social service provision and illustrate the boundary problems when trying to allocate people to be cared for by either the social or health care systems.

Table 5.18 Eligibility for care: case profiles: those thought in need of domiciliary care[a]

Case number	Profiles
2	An 87-year-old widow, lives alone and is newly discharged from hospital after a fall. She is increasingly frail and having difficulty walking because of severe arthritis. She manages most household tasks herself but was having difficulty with lifting and carrying. She needs help with cleaning and laundry. This is typical of referrals for help with domestic tasks
	Actual outcome: refused home care
6	Widow aged 91 years, lives alone and is newly discharged after cataract operation. Needs help with shopping and cleaning for limited four week period. This illustrates the types of short-term postoperative care needs resulting from a short hospital stay. Previously such patients might have remained in hospital until they could manage at home.
	Actual outcome: refused service as did not meet eligibility criteria
7	86-year-old widower, lives alone, but friendly neighbours drop in. Partially sighted, restricted mobility but can wash and dress himself. Needs help with cleaning, shopping and pension collection. This case indicates a 'typical' referral from concerned members of community who think this person should receive help.
	Actual outcome: given home care once a week but service withdrawn when eligibility criteria tightened
10	An 84-year-old, frail widow with mobility problems. Lives alone and has no regular support. Needs help to wash, dress, bathe, prepare food, and with shopping and the commode. This illustrates a person with considerable care needs. Unless these are meet she is 'at risk' of entry into care.
	Actual outcome: offered daily home care.

[a]Derived from: ACC/AMA, 1995

The resources allocated to the four case studies were very limited, reflecting the low level of service provision which is received by many clients of the community care system. For three of the case profiles, the majority of local authorities would be spending under £20 a week on their care. The situation was somewhat different for case profile 10. In this instance significant resources were being expended on the home care received by this person. The majority of local authorities surveyed (61.8%) reported that they would spend £60–140 a week on the care of this individual.

Table 5.19 Eligibility of case profiles for home care[a]

Case profile		Percentage local authorities reporting case profiles eligible for service		
	All	London	Metropolitan districts	Shire counties
2	83.8	94.4	87.5	76.3
6	87.5	88.2	100.0	79.5
7	79.7	88.2	87.5	71.1
10	98.8	94.7	100.0	100.0
n		18.0	24.0	38.0

[a]Derived from: ACC/AMA, 1995, Tables 2 and 3

Table 5.20 Provision of home care to case profiles[a]

	Cases			
	2	6	7	10
Local authorities: allocating home care (%)	97.0	98.6	100.0	89.4
allocating under 2 hrs home care (%)	47.7	56.6	73.0	1.3
allocating 5+ hrs home care (%)	15.4	7.2	1.6	97.4
spending under £20 on home care (%)	60.0	62.3	77.7	1.3

[a]Derived from: AAC/AMA, 1995, Tables 9, 10 and 11

Overall, these case profiles highlight several general issues regarding the implementation of community care. From the responses received there was a considerable degree of agreement about who was eligible for community care and the type of care required. The divergence emerged in the amount of home care which would be provided. From the survey it is not possible to determine why this variation emerged. However it is likely that it reflects: variations in the resources available to different local authorities; and differences between local authorities in the way that they target resources on 'high' need cases or spread them more generally (or indeed some combination of the two). A further interesting point emerges from this study. The theoretical resources allocated to these four case profiles was largely minimal. However, to fund one nursing home place at, for example, £200 a week, then services would have to be withdrawn from 10 people. This illustrates the conflict in demands and allocation of resources with which local authorities now have to cope routinely.

THE RELATIONSHIP BETWEEN FORMAL SERVICES AND INFORMAL CARERS

The very major contribution which the informal care sector makes to the maintenance of older people in the community has already been noted and will be examined in detail (Chapter 6). In this sector we examine the relative contributions these two sectors make to caring for older people in the community.

The contribution of informal carers and formal services

So far we have identified the extent of informal care provision and described the number and characteristics of older people receiving formal services which may be provided from a variety of sources (local authority, private contractor or voluntary agency). However these data only hint at the relative contribution of these different sources. One way of assessing this is to identify where people who need help with specific activities (such as personal or domestic care) actually receive this. This then enables us to evaluate the different contributions made by the various sectors.

Table 5.21 Who provides help for those aged 65 years and over needing help with locomotion/self care tasks? Great Britain, 1991[a]

| | Percentage receiving help – age (years) | | | |
| | 65–74 | | 75+ | |
	M	F	M	F
No-one	16	5	7	8
Spouse	71	46	52	15
Child	4	35	28	54
Other relative	4	16	17	15
Friend/neighbour	10	5	9	19
State service	6	13	19	17
Other	6	5	6	8

[a]Derived from: Goddard and Savage, 1994, Table 37

Using data from the 1991 GHS, Tables 5.21 and 5.22 indicate the sources of help given to older people who needed help with locomotion and self-care tasks and domestic tasks. Data are used from the 1991 GHS, in preference to the 1994 supplement, as the latter did not include the category of 'no help received' in the published tabulations. Hence, from the 1994 data it is not possible to estimate unmet need. Two main points are evident. First, it is the informal sector which is the largest provider of help to older people as far as these tasks are concerned. In both of these cases statutory services are not major contributors of care, even for the very old or those living alone. If we take a more detailed 'task orientated' approach this clarifies the relative contributions of the state, voluntary and informal care sectors (Table 5.23). With the exception of cutting toenails, which appears to be the almost exclusive activity of chiropodists, state services are the usual source of help for only a minority of older people. These data confirm that, with the exception of a few very specific tasks, it is the informal sector which is the main provider of help for older people.

Table 5.22 Who provides help for those aged 65 years and over needing help with domestic tasks? Great Britain, 1991[a]

| | Percentage receiving help – age (years) | | | |
| | 65–74 | | 75+ | |
	M	F	M	F
No-one	1	1	1	2
Spouse	53	41	39	154
Child	194	42	40	54
Other relative	15	16	20	21
Friend/neighbour	12	7	20	18
State service	18	16	23	26
Other	10	9	13	21

[a]Derived from: Goddard and Savage, 1994, Table 48

Table 5.23 Usual source of help for those unable to perform specific tasks alone: Great Britain, 1994[a]

| | Percentage receiving help from each source | | | |
	Locomotion/ self-care	Cut toenails	Bathing	Domestic
Spouse/partner	66	12	41	52
Other household	20	3	10	13
Non-house relative	7	5	21	28
Friend/neighbour	1	1	2	10
Voluntary worker	0	0	0	1
NHS social services	11	2	22	8
Paid help	0	0	1	12
Chiropodist	0	77	0	0
Other	0	0	2	1

[a]Derived from: GHS, 1996, Table 6.35

Second, there are a minority of people who reported that they needed help with these tasks but none was forthcoming. This was a larger problem for locomotion/self-care tasks than it was for domestic care. This may reflect the fact that it is easier to get friends, neighbours or more distant relatives to help with house cleaning and maintenance than with more personal care tasks such as dressing or washing. We can estimate the number of older people who need help and who report that they are not receiving it. This estimate suggest that approximately a quarter of a million older people (230 000) need help with domestic/personal care tasks which they are not receiving. Hence there remains a substantial amount of unmet need in the community. If we apply these prevalence estimates to the county of Surrey, this suggests that there are 1976 people aged 65 years and over in the county who are not receiving the help that they need with locomotion/self care tasks and 406 who have an unmet need for domestic help. The extent of the potential unmet need among older people living in the community is indicated by Bowling *et al.* (1993). They note that the answers given to questions about unmet need depend upon how the question is posed. Asked directly if they wanted additional services, e.g. district nursing, few responded 'yes' to this type of question (the only exception being chiropody for which up to 22% wanted this service). However, when asked about difficulties experience with activities of daily living and the need for more help to cope with this, 45% at follow-up (37% at baseline) reported unmet need. When asked about the source of such help, 88% expressed a preference for 'professional' (health/social service) help rather than family/friends (6%) or private/voluntary services (2%).

CONCLUSION

In this chapter we have looked at the role of the formal service sector in maintaining older people in the community. It is evident that older people remain the main user group for all the main health and social care system. However it still remains unclear as to which models of care would be the most appropriate for enabling older people to remain at home for as long as possible. The increased and expected role of the independent sector in domiciliary care provision is starting to emerge. However it is not clear that a quasi market in health and social care will actually increase the range and quality of services being provided for older people (or indeed other client groups).

While the provision of services has increased the actual percentage of older people being supported shows little change. There is, to date, little evidence of services being more effectively 'targeted' at those 'most in need' or that packages of care tailor made to meet individual needs are emerging on a significant scale. What is certain is that there remain considerable unmet needs among older people in the community and that the informal care sector is absolutely vital in maintaining older people in the community. One of the challenges which faces the successful implementation of community care is the need for the formal and informal sectors to develop effective ways of working together. Twigg (1992) has argued that carers occupy an ambiguous location in the social care system and that it is difficult to determine what the 'proper' relationship should be. She has developed a four-fold typology to describe the relationship.

- Carers as resources. In this scenario informal care provides the 'taken for granted' context with services concentrating upon the client's needs.
- Carers as co-workers. Here the aim is to integrate formal services with the contribution of the informal.
- Carers as co-clients. Here, carers are seen as clients in their own right, and services are aimed at improving their circumstances.
- Superseded carers. Here the emphasis is upon 'freeing' the dependent older person from the 'dependent' relationship upon the carers and is most influential in the care of adults with learning disabilities.

Twigg (1992) notes that the relationship between carers and formal services changes and may illustrate several of the models described above at different times. As yet the relationship between carers and the formal services remains problematic. One of the problems is that carers are usually referred to as a single group. This implies an homogeneous profile and a single set of needs. In the next chapter we will consider in more detail the nature of informal care provision and highlight the diversity of different groups and situations covered by this single umbrella term.

6

Care by the community

INTRODUCTION

Just as community care was not 'invented' in 1993 nor was the informal provision of care for older people by family, friends and neighbours 'invented' in the 1980s. It seems highly likely that it has always been the informal sector (family, friends and neighbours) who have provided the bulk of care to those with long-term health problems. This expectation was enshrined in the 1930 Poor Law Act which stated: 'It should be the duty of the father, grandfather, mother, grandmother, husband or child of a poor, old, blind, lame or impotent person, or other poor person, not able to work, if possessed of sufficient means, to relieve and maintain that person not able to work.' (Means and Smith, 1994, p. 19). However it was in the 1980s that a now significant body of research started to identify the true extent of the informal care sector. It carefully enumerated the characteristics of those who provided such care, who they provided it to and how much care was provided. This chapter explores the contribution of the informal sector and considers the nature and characteristics of those who provide informal care. We will try to examine if the provision of care by informal carers has increased (or decreased) with the development of the modern welfare state and consider how carers perceive their role and the implementation of the community care policy. We conclude with a consideration of general attitudes towards caring and the role of the formal and informal sectors.

WHAT IS THE INFORMAL CARE SECTOR?

The provision of care to older people is divided, but not equally (Chapter 5), between the formal and informal sectors. The potential and contribution of the informal sector is recognized in recent policy development in so far as documents refer constantly to 'users' and carers'. However, they rarely distinguish between the two or recognize that the needs of these two parties are not necessarily synonymous. Carers are now entitled to a community care assessment in their own right. However, given the large number of carers, this has significant resource implications even if no services are supplied after the assessment. Typically, carers are referred to as if they constitute a unitary social group with identical needs. In this chapter we will be attempting to disaggregate the social group 'carers' and consider the homogeneity (or otherwise) of this very important group, without the support of whom the policy of community care is ultimately doomed to failure.

The first question we need to answer is one of definition. What is the informal care sector? Who is a carer? The informal sector may be defined as care provided by family, friends and neighbours which is not organized through a statutory or voluntary agency. Typically such care is not provided for money but rather stems from the complex relationships of responsibilities and obligations which arise within families (Finch, 1995). The informal sector has always been the main provider of help to older people, especially with the non-professional, 'non-specialist' personal and household tasks which are required to maintain them in the community. As we have already seen this statement is applicable to the contemporary period contradicting the powerful popular myth that older people are neglected by their family and that the main burden of caring for older people falls upon the state.

The importance of the informal sector in maintaining older people in the community (and indeed other groups with long-term care needs) is now an accepted and acknowledged part of community care policy. Indeed the key role of informal carers was acknowledged in the Griffiths White Paper (1988) which stated: '... the reality is that most care is provided by family, friends and neighbours'. Implicit within this statement is the notion of 'carers as a resource' as proposed by Twigg (1992), and an assumption that state services will not be forthcoming until the informal network is exhausted or non-existent. This quotation implies the existence of a wide network of potential carers living in the community, and suggests that a variety of different individuals (relatives, friends, neighbours) could be involved in the care of an older person. As we shall see later in this chapter the situation does not match up to the idealistic expectations of policy makers.

WHAT IS A CARER?

The term 'carer' now has widespread currency in academic, lay and policy making circles. However, it is not easy to produce a definition of a carer. Initially, research in this field was dominated by small qualitative studies in which carers were self-identified (Ungerson, 1987; Nissel and Bonnerjea, 1982; Lewis and Meredith, 1988). Such studies helped raise the profile of carers and served to shed light on the daily experience of carers. Much of this agenda setting research grew out of feminist concern for the 'oppression' of women within the family arising from child care and later caring for elderly parents (in law). As such it identified the 'burden' caring placed upon women because of restricted employment opportunities and health problems (Twigg, 1992). The work by Brody (1981) emphasized the importance of 'women in the middle' in the provision of care of older relatives; these are middle-aged women who, having discharged their child care responsibilities, are then faced with accepting responsibility for the care of an aged parent.

These and other authors help to generate interest in the topic of informal care. However the strongly feminist orientation of the initial researchers influenced the type of research questions posed and the methodologies used to answer them. For example, the identification and selection of samples for study meant that it was often difficult to draw general conclusions from the stimulating results produced. Similarly such research focused exclusively upon women as carers and did not acknowledge the potential contribution that men could make in this area (Arber and Gilbert, 1989).

The survey of carers included as part of the 1985 GHS (Green 1988), was an attempt to undertake a large scale nationally representative prevalence type survey of the provision of informal care within Great Britain. The survey was repeated in 1990 (OPCS, 1992). The definition used in these studies, which asked about extra family responsibilities resulting from the care of someone who was elderly (or sick or handicapped), is shown in Table 6.1. In 1985, this definition results in 14% of the adult population defining themselves as a carer (12% of males and 15% of females); this percentage had increased to 14% and 17% respectively in the 1990 survey (Arber and Ginn, 1995).

Table 6.1 Prevalence of caring among the adult population (aged 16+) – the 1985 and 1990 GHS surveys[a]

| | *Percentage defining themselves as carers* | | | | | |
| | *1985* | | | *1990* | | |
	M	F	All	M	F	All
a) Co-resident care Some people have *extra family* responsibilities because they look after someone who is sick, handicapped or elderly – Is there anyone living with you who is sick, handicapped or elderly whom you look after or give special help to?	2	2	2	4	4	4
b) Extra-resident care And how about people not living with you, do you provide some regular source of help for any sick, handicapped or elderly relative, friend or neighbour not living with you?	10	7	9	10	13	12
Total percentage of adults who define themselves as carers	12	9	10	14	17	16

[a]Derived from: Arber and Ginn, 1991 and 1995

Interpreting this apparent increase in the prevalence of caring is problematic. It may indeed represent a 'real' increase in the percentage of the population becoming a carer over this time frame. However, one criticism that has been levelled at the GHS carer definition is that it is understood differently by men and women. It is argued that women see caring as part of their 'normal' responsibilities and hence do not define themselves as a carer. Alternatively we may speculate that the increased prevalence of caring apparent in Table 6.1 (especially among women) may result from a decreased willingness of women responders to see caring as part of 'normal' family life and being more willing to define themselves as a carer, perhaps in response to the greater public awareness of carers.

How do members of the general population understand the term 'carers' which is used so widely in almost all community care documentation and information. Of the general population only 5% think a carer is someone who looks after a family member or friend who cannot look after themselves because of frailty, disability or illness (CNA,1996). The other main definitions of a 'carer' identified in the CNA survey (CNA, 1996) were someone with a *paid* job involving caring/working for social services sources (31%), a voluntary worker (7%), or a 'caring' person 79% (the remaining respondents didn't know). However the CNA (1996) survey does provide some apparent validity for the GHS data as using the CNA definition of a carer as 'someone who looks after a family member or friend who cannot look after themselves because of frailty, disability or illness' 12% of the adult population (11% males and 13% females) self-defined themselves as carers.

Typology of caring

As noted above, the GHS (Green, 1988) reported that 10% of the adult population (i.e. those aged 16 years and over) defined themselves as carers. Applied to the general population this estimate suggests that 6 million adults in Great Britain (or 6.8 million using the 1990 estimate of 15%) are actively engaged in 'looking after or providing some regular service for someone who was sick, elderly or handicapped' either in their own household or elsewhere.

This large scale estimate of the number of carers within the population was treated uncritically by both organizations representing the views of carers and the DoH. How accurate is this estimate and what are the main characteristics of 'carers'? Although a large percentage of the population self-identified themselves as carers detailed analysis reveals that those heavily involved in caring may be considerably less than the initial estimate. Analysis of the OPCS survey of the prevalence of disability among adults and children suggests that there are 1.3 million 'main carers', that is individuals who spent most of their time caring, in Britain (Parker, 1990). How can these discrepant estimates of the number of informal carers from three different surveys be reconciled?

The differences between the estimates relates to the different definitions used to identify carers. These relate to three main factors: the household relationship between carer and dependent person; the carer's level of responsibility for their dependent, and; the type of caring activity. Each of these approaches is considered below.

Co-resident and extra-resident carers

Arber and Ginn (1990, 1991, 1995) have concentrated upon those caring for elderly people. Their analysis has distinguished between carers who live with the person for whom they are caring (co-resident carers) and those looking after someone in a different household (extra-resident carers). They argue that provision of informal care within the same household is fundamentally different from extra-resident care and that in policy terms the two types of caring situation should not be treated as the same. Care within the same household is primarily for parents and spouses whereas extra-resident care is received by more distant relatives and friends/neighbours (Table 6.2). These authors also analysed the amount of time spent caring. This revealed that, on average in 1985, co-resident carers spent 53 hours a week of care compared with nine hours for extra-resident carers (Arber and Ginn, 1991). In 1990 over 50% of co-resident carers spent 35 hours a week or more caring (Arber and Ginn, 1995). Clearly co-resident carers are providing a different level of care and support and represent different needs for support from the formal sector than do those who are extra-resident carers. We may speculate that it is those who are receiving intensive informal care who are the ones who are 'at risk' of admission to nursing/residential care.

Table 6.2 Characteristics of informal care provision to older people by type of carer[a]

Dependent	Co-resident carer	Extra-resident carer
Spouse	40	-
Parent	36	39
Parent in law	11	15
Other relative	18	18
Friend/neighbour	-	27
Total number of hours of informal care provided (%)	61	39

[a]Derived from: Arber and Ginn, 1991, Table 8.2

The network of informal care?

Evandrou (1991) concentrated upon the carers level of responsibility for their dependent as the distinguishing characteristic of different type of carers. She identifies three different types of carers; sole carers, joint carers (where the caring responsibility is borne jointly with another person and peripheral carers (i.e. where there are more than two people providing care; this might approximate to the network of informal care which was referred to in the Griffiths report). The majority of carers in the 1985 GHS survey (54%) were sole carers, 11% were joint carers and 35% were peripheral carers. Hence, for the majority of dependents (whatever their age), there is only a very limited network of people involved in their care. While the contribution of the informal sector is hugely significant most of it is being provided by a sole carer.

Caring activities

Parker and Lawton (1994) have developed a typology based upon the activities of caring. This defines carers on the basis of what they do rather than who they are, who they help or the number of other carers involved in caring. It is, perhaps, more useful from a policy development and community care perspective to discuss caring from the perspective of what is being done. Although it is useful to know who carers are and how many others are involved, it is not possible to develop services which support carers if the types of caring being provided is unknown. Without such information we might develop gardening services when carers are busy cutting their dependents toenails (or vice versa). The typology developed by Parker and Lawton (1994) is based upon the eight caring tasks included in the GHS survey. This of course limits the development of their theoretical model as they are confined to the topics covered in the survey. These are shown in Table 6.3 which shows that some caring tasks, such as practical help (e.g. shopping preparing meals) were much more common than other tasks, such as physical care or giving medicines. Clearly there is some overlap between the tasks and this formed the basis for the sixfold typology they developed (Table 6.4). The most common form of caring was the provision of practical help which was received by 50% of those receiving care.

Table 6.3 The prevalence of different types of caring tasks: Great Britain, 1995[a]

Task	Percentage of all carers undertaking this task
Personal care	22
Physical care	20
Paperwork	39
Practical	82
Keeping company	64
Taking out	48
Giving medicine	20
Keeping an eye on	71

[a]Derived from: Lawton and Parker, 1994, Table 2.1

Table 6.4 A typology of caring tasks[a]

Category	Carers performing (%)	Estimated percentage of adults
Personal and physical care	12	1.7
Personal not physical care	9	1.3
Physical not personal care	8	1.1
Other practical help	50	6.9
Practical help only	8	1.1
Other	14	1.9

[a]Derived from: Parker and Lawton, 1994, Table 2.3; and Parker, 1992, Table 1.2

Like the previous two ways of looking at carers this task orientated approach distinguishes between those who provide a limited amount of care and those with extensive caring responsibilities. Of those providing personal and physical help 80% were sole carers and 69% were living in the same household as their dependents.

Each of the definitions of caring considered previously can, therefore, be refined to yield a firm definition of those who are actively involved in the care and maintenance of frail vulnerable people in the community. One of the problems with the GHS is that these definitions apply to all carers not simply those caring for older people. However as at least 75% of those receiving care in the GHS samples are aged 65 years and over this is not a major limitation.

Estimating the number of carers

Using the different approaches to the definition and classification of carers we can estimate the number and percentage of adults involved in the provision of informal care both nationally and locally (Table 6.5). Three definitions (co-resident caring, caring for over 20 hours a week and providing personal and physical care) yield very similar prevalence rates, and it seems most helpful from the community care perspective to use one of these in estimating the number of informal carers within a specific locality. However the sole carer category is too gross and needs to be refined to sole co-resident care.

Table 6.5 Estimating the number of carers nationally and locally[a]

Type of carer	Estimated adult population (%)	Estimated number - nationally	Estimated number in Surrey
Provides personal and physical care	1.7	766 649	13 939
Co-resident carer	2.0	901 940	16 399
Caring for 20 hours a week	3.0	1 352 910	24 598
Sole carer	8.0	3 607 760	65 595
Sole co-resident carer	1.6		

[a]Number of adults in GB in 1994: 45 097 000
Number of adults in Surrey in 1994: 819 940

WHO IS A CARER?

As we noted earlier perhaps the most influential factor in the 'discovery' of informal care has been feminism. In the 1980s a feminist critique of community care developed (Land, 1978; Finch and Groves, 1980; 1983; Ungerson, 1987; Dally, 1988). This argued that social policies, such as community care, contained implicit assumptions that caring was almost exclusively a task undertaken by women who were usually daughters (in law) caring for their parents (in law).

However analysis of the 1985 and 1990 GHS surveys has revealed that the characteristics of those with caring responsibilities do not neatly fit into the feminist stereotype. Like the different ways of defining and categorizing carers so the characteristics of those providing care are not homogenous. Carers, even within the more rigorously defined groups identified earlier, like many other subsets of the general population, are a heterogenous group. Their needs for support and services will vary according to their own characteristics, the type of care provided, the involvement of others in the provision of care and the situation in which they are providing care.

The discovery of the male carer

One of the more challenging findings from the GHS surveys has been the 'discovery' of male carers (Arber and Gilbert, 1989; Arber and Ginn, 1995). As noted earlier, approximately 10% of adult males defined themselves as extra-resident carers and 4% (2% in 1985) as co-resident carers. Consequently the role of the male carer is now acknowledged and discussed (Evandrou,1991; Parker and Lawton, 1994; Rose and Bruce, 1995; Wilson, 1995).

However the analysis of both the location of care provided and the type of care provided shows the complexity of the gender differences in informal caring. Where care is being provided to someone in the same household then carers are almost equally divided between males and females (40% and 60% respectively in 1985, and 45% and 55% respectively in 1990) (Arber and Ginn, 1991; 1995). However, when care is received outside the household, then the majority of carers are women (69% in 1985, and 62% in 1990) (Arber and Ginn, 1991;1995). So, although male carers are important, they are usually confined to a specific caring situation; that of a co-resident carer usually looking after an elderly spouse. Arber and Ginn (1995) argue that for women (but not men) marriage defines them as the (potential) carer of anyone within the household; men are seen as only having limited caring responsibilities beyond their spouse.

How does the prevalence of caring vary with age?

Including both co-resident and extra-resident carers Table 6.6 identifies the peak age for caring as 45–59 years. However one important feature illustrated is the contribution of older people themselves to the care of elderly people within the community; 17% of those aged 60–74 years and 8% of those aged 75 years and over self-identified themselves as carers. Aggregating this to the situation of Great Britain then at least 1 166 880 people aged 65 years and over (women and men) are carers. This is reinforced by the 1990 GHS which found that 15% of people over 60 years of age were caring for a sick, elderly or handicapped person compared with 16% aged 16–59 years (Table 6.7). This starkly contradicts the popular stereotype of older people as a dependent group making little contribution to the wellbeing of the nation as a whole. Disregarding any other contribution they may make to family life (such as the care of grand/great-grandchildren) older people are clearly important contributors to the care of older people.

Table 6.6 Percentage of adults who are carers by age and sex: Great Britain, 1985a

Age	Male	Female	Total
16–29	6	7	8
30–44	10	16	14
45–59	16	24	21
60–74	14	18	17
75+	10	6	8

[a]Derived from: Evandrou, 1991, Table 1

Table 6.7 Prevalence of caring and extra household help by older people: Great Britain, 1990[a]

Age	Co-resident carer (%)		Extra-resident carer (%)		Regular help to someone outside (%)	
	M	F	M	F	M	F
60–64	6	6	13	17	-	-
65–69	5	6	10	10	46	46
70–74	8	6	9	8	37	33
75–79	6	5	5	10	30	22
80+	8	2	3	2	16	10
All 60+	6	5	9	10	-	-
All 16–59	3	3	10	15	-	-

[a]Derived from: Jarvis *et al.*, 1996, Table 6 and Figures 5.6 and 5.2

Overall one-fifth of all carers are aged over 65 years. Older carers represent 26% of all co-resident carers, 15% of extra-resident carers, 21% of main carers and 27% of those caring for over 20 hours a week (Green, 1988). The contribution of older people within society is emphasized by the fact that, according to the 1990 GHS, 35% of men aged 65 years and over and 29% of women 'gave help to someone living outside their household' (Table 6.7). However older carers are much more likely to be providing care to someone within their own household than younger carers. This reflects the fact that, for older people, it is for their spouse that they are caring (Arber and Gilbert, 1989).

Where care is being provided by women aged 45–64 years then this consists largely of women caring for their parents (in law). These are two totally different situations which present different problems and require different policy responses. Hence it is quite erroneous to develop policy which does not recognize these fundamental differences.

Of those aged 16–64 years identified as carers in the 1985 GHS 11% reported that they were working full-time and 18% worked part-time (Green, 1988). There was no variation in the percentage reporting themselves as carers between manual (14%) and non-manual workers (14%). Indeed there were very little socio-economic status variations between different types of carers. We will consider the labour market participation of carers further in the section looking at the consequences of becoming a carer. One variable which has been lacking in this analysis is that of ethnicity. We know very little about the extent and nature of informal care provision within Britain's ethnic minority populations. Blakemore and Boneham (1994) draw attention to our stereotypical view of minority elders being embedded in a close knit and caring family. However this fails to take account of variations between different minority communities (e.g. treating members of Chinese, Afro-Caribbean and Asian communities as if they were a single group; clearly an error of judgement) and the fact that because these individuals are mostly migrants and may be separated from their extended family and may only be members of very small family networks in the UK. However, with the 'ageing' of our minority communities this is going to become a topic of considerable policy relevance and one which researchers should start to examine seriously.

WHY DO PEOPLE CARE?

We have expended considerable effort on quantifying the extent, type and consequences of providing informal care. Rather less attention has been given to considering the question 'why people care'. The provision of care in the informal or family situation is clearly a result of the inter-relationship between a variety of factors. Caring takes place in a relationship between the carer and his/her dependent that has developed over a number of years and which is embedded in a web of family and community responsibilities. Parker (1990) distinguished between caring (as in being concerned about someone) and tending (i.e. performing tasks to look after them). In the debate about informal care the focus has been upon tending (i.e. doing things for people that they cannot do for themselves). However interpretation of caring and distinguishing where caring starts and the 'normal' family pattern of tending stops is problematic.

Finch (1995) has undertaken one of the few studies examining the nature of obligations and responsibilities within families concentrating upon the adult child–parent relationship rather than marital relationships. Finch (1989) has identified a hierarchy of caring obligations. She suggests that informal care is organized around four central relationships.

- The marital relationship is of primary importance so that the spouse is the first source of care for married people.
- The parent–child relationship is the second source of obligation. Children

become a principal source of care for elderly parents, and parents the main source of care for disabled children.

- Those who share a household are major care providers; the child who shares the parental home is more likely to provide care than siblings living away from home.
- Where there is a 'choice' between male and female relatives as to who becomes the carer, then it is the female relative who usually becomes the carer.

Finch (1995) argues that the spouse and child–parent caring relationships are arrived at by differing routes. The marital relationship is qualitatively different from that of parents and children. Marriage is a legally contracted relationship, based upon a promise of mutual care and support and the establishment of a shared household. As such, becoming the carer of a disabled spouse may be perceived as an integral part of the relationship and consequently may be 'assumed' by policy makers as a given fact. However there is clearly more scope for looking at the meaning of long-term marriage, the relationships between the partners and their expectations (Askham,1995; Wilson, 1995).

Finch (1995) argues that filial responsibilities are not based upon fixed obligations but upon commitments and reciprocal relationships developed over time between parents and their adult children. Thus, perceived responsibilities for caring for their parents will depend very much upon the relationships within the family. As such this means that policy makers cannot make clear assumptions about the willingness (or otherwise) of adult children to care for their parents. This would suggest that the provision of informal care outside the family/kinship obligations identified above would be comparatively rare and confined to less 'personal' tasks. Table 6.2 indicates that the majority of care is indeed received by close family members (i.e. spouse or parent (in law)). Although 22% of care givers are looking after a friend/neighbour, this represents only 7% of total time caring as compared with 81% for close family members (30% for spouse, 40% for parent and 11% for a parent-in-law) (Arber and Ginn, 1991).

WHO IS BEING CARED FOR?

From the perspective of community care policy we need to know both who is doing the caring and who is being cared for. Consequently most studies of informal care include a profile of those who are being cared for; the recipients of care. The demographic profile of dependents, or receivers of informal care, from three studies of informal caring are shown in Table 6.8. All three studies illustrate that it is women who constitute the majority of those receiving informal care and that the majority of recipients are people aged 65 years and over (ranging from 76% in the 1985 GHS study (Green, 1988) to 55% in the 1996 CNA study). These differences reflect the different types of study; one is attempting to present a 'national' survey of the nature of informal care provision (the GHS survey) while the other is based upon data provided from members of the CNA and it is highly likely that members of that organization are not representative of 'all' carers (although this does not detract from the quality of the data it does make it less representative). Indeed it would seem that members of the CNA are more likely than the general population of carers to be looking after a younger dependent. This may reflect the fact the older carers are less likely to define themselves as 'a carer' (but rather see their caring role as an extension of their role of spouse) and so would not join such an organization.

Table 6.8 Who is being cared for (%): a comparison of several surveys[a]

Characteristics of dependent	GHS 1985	CNA 1992	CNA 1996
Male (%)	30	19	n/a
Under 16	3	8	6
16–64	21	29	39
65+	76	63	55

[a]Derived from: GHS: Green, 1988; CNA, 1992 and 1996

Table 6.9 Disability of carers dependents (%): a comparison of the 1985 GHS and CNA surveys[a]

Type of disability	Dependents with disability (%)	
	GHS 1985	CNA 1992
Physical	73	44
Mental	5	19
Mental and physical	16	-
Old age	4	29
Learning	-	7
Other	2	-

[a]Derived from: GHS: Green, 1988; CNA, 1992

Large scale surveys of carers do not reveal much about the nature of the disabilities or health problems which their dependents experience. Table 6.9 compares the results of two surveys which suggest that the majority of dependents have problems with physical disability while a significant minority, approximately 20%, are mentally frail (presumably because of dementia, although this is not actually stated). Overall, the majority of carers (69%) are looking after a physically frail person aged over 65 years. Carers looking after a person living with them were more likely to be looking after a mentally frail person (31%) than carers who were not co-resident (17%).

What do carers do?

Evidence documenting the contribution of carers may be derived from both large scale surveys and more detailed qualitative investigations. Consistently large studies have indicated the diversity of tasks undertaken by carers. Table 6.10 indicates that the provision of practical help is the most often provided type of care. However the type of care provided varies markedly between co-resident and extra-resident carers. Co-resident people are characterized by high levels of provision of personal and physical help which is much less commonly provided by extra resident carers. Help with personal care is most likely to be received by co-resident dependents aged 65 years and over; 64% of dependents in this category received help with personal care compared with 41% of dependents aged 16–29 years. Women carers are much more likely to be involved in providing personal care than males (Table 6.10) (Arber and Ginn, 1995).

Table 6.10 Types of help given by different types of carers (%): Great Britain, 1985[a]

| | Percentage of carers providing | | | | | |
| | Co-resident | | Extra-resident | | All carers | |
	M	F	M	F	M	F
Personal care	43	62	7	16	19	28
Giving medicine	37	53	10	14	19	24
Physical help	46	46	10	14	22	22
Paperwork	42	51	40	36	41	40
Other practical	82	80	82	82	82	82
Keeping company	63	64	63	69	63	68
Taking out	60	49	50	46	53	47
Keeping eye on	75	83	63	72	67	75

[a]Derived from: Green, 1988, Table 4.20

The provision of such tasks is usually being provided on a regular basis (CNA, 1996). The 1985 GHS (Green, 1988) reported that, overall, 40% of carers provided care for up to two days a week and 40% for seven days a week (Green, 1988). However, the level of commitment to the provision of informal care shows the by now familiar distinction between co-resident and extra-resident carers. This reveals that 92% of co-resident carers looked after their dependant seven days a week compared with 18% of extra-resident carers (Green, 1988). This is reflected in the number of hours carers spend caring for their dependent. Almost half of co-resident carers (45%) spend over 50 hours a week caring compared with under 1% of extra-resident carers and 14% of all carers (Green, 1988). Older carers (i.e. those aged 65 years and over) who are co-resident carers are the group most likely to be caring for over 50 hours a week. Almost two-thirds (59%) of all co-resident carers aged 65 years and over are caring for more than 50 hours compared with 38% of carers aged 30–44 years (Green, 1988). This serves to reinforce the earlier comment about the extensive nature of the contribution towards informal care, and community care more generally, made by older people themselves.

Providing informal care is not a short term commitment. In the 1985 GHS survey (Green, 1988) while 13% of carers had been doing this for less than a year, 43% had been caring for more than five years (Table 6.11). However we should be slightly cautious in interpreting this table as any cross-sectional study will over-emphasize those long-term carers and under-estimate the number of short term carers. Again co-resident carers were the most likely to have been a 'long-term' carer (i.e. for five years or longer) than extra-resident carers (55% compared to 39%).

Table 6.11 Number of years caring by type of carer (%): Great Britain, 1985[a]

| | Percentage of carers | | |
	Co-resident carer	Extra-resident carer	All
Under 1 year	9	14	13
1–2 years	19	28	25
3–4 years	18	19	19
5+ years	55	39	43

[a]Derived from: Green, 1988, Table 4.16

Becoming a carer

One of the issues noted earlier was the definition of 'a carer' and the likelihood that women would be less likely to self-define themselves as a carer as compared with men. There is little research looking at how people become carers and how they then come to accept this label. Research carried out with members of the CNA provides some insight into how carers come to perceive themselves as undertaking this role (CNA, 1992). This study revealed that only one-third of their members realized immediately that they were taking on this role, while 14% took 10 years to realize they had undertaken this role. This highlights the fact that many carers do not accept that they are undertaking this role but merely see themselves as fulfilling 'normal' family/domestic responsibilities. As such they may be reluctant to seek help or accept the label of 'carers' offered to them by professional and voluntary agencies.

What led to carers recognizing that they were indeed 'carers'? In the majority of people who responded to the CNA survey 53% of carers reported that it was contact with a health/social services professional which resulted in them feeling that they were a carer. Family (26%), the media (17%) and contact with the CNA (24%) were important factors in making people feel that they were carers.

In the majority of cases included in the CNA study (79%), the carers felt they had no choice in taking on the caring role. This was particularly true for those caring for a spouse (86%) or other relative (78%) as compared to those looking after non-relatives (47%). Three main reasons explained why people had undertaken the caring role: duty (reported by 32%), the nature of their relationship to the dependent person (38%) and lack of any alternative (34%). For a significant number of carers their relationship with the dependent was sufficient to explain why they had become a carer. This was typified by such comments as 'the person I care for is my husband', 'because she's my wife' and 'as it was my husband who had the stroke, I became the carer – if it had been the other way about he'd have been the carer'. These quotations seem to fit with the model proposed by Finch (1995) that caring for a spouse is seen as part of the obligations of the role of husband/wife.

The lack of viable care alternatives, a rather negative reason, was also an important stimulus to becoming a carer as typified by the comment 'mother won't go into a home'. Duty, or perhaps obligation, is a less 'coercive' term and was the other main stimulus to care. This was indicated by such comments as 'it didn't occur to me that it wasn't my responsibility' and 'it seems natural – I've never thought of myself as a carer until recently'. Although the CNA (1992) survey did identify some examples of people feeling 'pressured' into becoming a carer, it seems that the majority of respondents in that study became carers willingly.

THE DYNAMICS OF CARING

The majority of the literature concerned with estimating the extent and nature of the provision of informal care have been cross sectional studies conducted at a single point in time (a point prevalence study). As such, these types of studies do not give any indication of the incidence of caring (i.e. how many 'new' carers take on the role in a given time period), over represent those who have been caring for extensive periods of time and tell us little about ex-carers (i.e. those who, for whatever reason, have given up their caring responsibility). As yet there are no large longitudinal studies which study the relevant history of the informal carer from the start of the commitment until its end. However some data are available about some of these issues notably the incidence of caring and ex-carers.

The incidence of caring

Data from the GHS survey (Green, 1988) indicate that 13% of carers had been caring for less than one year; 9% of co-resident carers and 14% of extra resident carers. This compares with 17% in the 1996 CNA survey and 3% in the 1992 survey. Applying this estimate to the general population, of the six million carers (estimated from the GHS) 780 000 of them are 'new' carers (i.e. they have become a carer within the last year). Taking the much more restricted definition of a carer as someone who is a co-resident carer, which represents about 1.2 million adults then 9% or 108 000 will have become carers in the last 12 months.

Stopping caring: becoming an ex-carer

Just as new carers are beginning to provide informal care so some carers are becoming ex-carers. Data from the CNA (1992) have data on 834 ex-carers in their survey, the majority of whom had stopped caring within the last two years. The main reason that carers had stopped caring was, not surprisingly, the death of their dependent (reported by 61% of ex-carers). The other main reason for them giving up their caring responsibilities was the admission of their dependent into a residential or nursing home (28%). In a very, very few instances another person had taken over the caring responsibility (reported by 1% of ex-carers).

These data, therefore indicate that once the role of carer is accepted then this is a long-term responsibility which is only discharged when the dependent dies or is admitted to long-term care. How does the loss of the caring role affect the carer? Of those included in the CNA survey, 43% reported that they experienced loneliness once they lost the role of carer. Other problems experienced included depression (37%), loss of income (31%), loss of friends (12%) and difficulties of getting paid work (9%). Not surprisingly, those caring for a spouse were the most likely to report these problems. The survey did not include any questions about how the loss of the caring role may have positively influenced their lives.

More data about the effect of becoming an ex-carer are reported by McLaughlin and Ritchie (1994). They followed up 157 ex-carers who had been receiving a carer benefit, invalid care allowance (ICA), and also undertook qualitative in-depth interviews with a small sample of carers. These authors adopted the typology of caring roles proposed by Lewis and Meredith (1988) in their study of daughters caring for mothers. They categorized their carers into three groups; balancing acts, integration and immersion. The consequences for ex-carers who had 'immersed' themselves in caring such that it provided their main sense of identity found the consequences of becoming an ex-carer more problematic than the other two categories, especially with reference to the social and psychological after-effects. However there is a clear need for more research which looks at the consequences for people of giving up caring.

THE CONSEQUENCES OF CARING

How does taking on the role of carer affect the lives of those who undertake this service? This is a difficult area to research as it covers a long-term or life course perspective of the financial, employment, health and social consequences of becoming a carer. However, as such data are unavailable, we have to use cross-sectional studies which compare the characteristics of carers with non-carers (or indeed we can compare non-carers with ex-carers). However the methodological limitations of this approach need to be borne in mind. For example a person with few qualifications and limited employment prospects may be more likely to become a carer than someone with better qualifications and prospects. However to draw the inference that it was 'caring' which was the 'cause' of their poor employment prospects would be erroneous. This highlights the problems involved in this type of analysis. If we show differences in, for example, the financial circumstances of non-carers, ex-carers and carers, we must be very cautious in attributing any identified differences to the effect of caring. The relationship is probably much more complex than one of simple cause and effect. In the next sections we will try to review the current situation regarding the employment, financial, health and social circumstances of carers as compared with non-carers. Where possible we will also make comparisons between the circumstances of ex-carers to try and establish the 'long-term' effects of being a carer.

The benefits of caring

We have already documented the extensive nature and commitment which characterizes the role of informal carer and have indicated that people undertake this role because of the strength of their relationship to the dependent. We have noted that there are some negative consequences which result from undertaking this role. However it is also important to determine the benefits and rewards of undertaking this task.

Grant and Nolan (1993) surveyed members of the CNA to look at sources of satisfaction among carers. In their sample of 671 carers, 60% gave answers to an 'open' question about sources of satisfaction derived from their role of carer. This level of satisfaction with 'caring' was somewhat lower than had been reported by Clifford (1990) who reported satisfaction levels of over 90%. However it is easy to see that it would be very easy for respondents to give what they thought was the correct, socially accepted response. Grant and Nolan's approach yielded 546 statements made by carers about the sources of satisfaction that they derived. These were classified into 14 main groups which were then grouped into three main categories.

- Satisfaction deriving from the relationship between carer and dependent. This was the largest group of comments and related to the satisfaction gained by carers from caring for their dependent and includes such things as altruism, reciprocity and the obligations deriving from marriage (e.g. 'what little I am able to do is for the love and vows I took with my wife, with no sense of duty' and 'For better or worse I fully believe in this' (Grant and Nolan, 1993, p. 153).
- Satisfaction derived by the carer – such as the development of a positive role, feeling useful and responding to new challenges.
- Satisfaction derived from the avoidance of negative consequences for the dependent. This is a rather perverse category which describes the satisfaction carers got from avoiding the entry into care of their dependent or the pride gained in offering higher quality/more tailored (or personalized) care than could be hoped for from the statutory sector.

Grant and Nolan (1993) report that satisfaction with the caring role did not vary between men and women or with level of dependency, but was highest among those caring for close family members (children/spouses/parents) rather than more distant relationships. Consequently they argue that satisfaction with the role of carer is related to the quality of the relationship between carer and dependent rather than more objective measures such as the level of disability of the person for whom they are caring. This suggests that interventions aimed at maintaining the quality of the relationship between carer and dependent could be effective in maintaining the role of informal carers. Clearly there is scope for more research looking at the motivations of carers and the evaluation of interventions designed to promote and strengthen informal care.

Employment

Given the demographic profile of informal carers with a substantial number being aged over 65 years, then participation in the formal labour market is not an option for a significant number of carers. In 1996, the CNA survey reported that 59% of their respondents were not employed. However this suggests that 40% of carers are both providers of informal care and actively engaged in the labour market. Looked at another way, the 1985 GHS survey (Green, 1988) revealed that 13% of employed adults were carers (11% males, 18% married women and 13% non-married women) (Evandrou, 1991). For men there was no difference in the prevalence of caring between full-time workers (11%) and part-time (under 23 hours a week) workers (12%) (Evandrou,1991). However for women there was a marked difference between full-time and part-time workers. Of married women, 20% of part-time workers were carers as compared with 13% of full-time workers; for married women the percentages were 17% and 10% respectively. However, as noted above, we must be cautious in drawing the inference that caring 'causes' women to work part-time. Over time, Joshi (1995) has noted that women's involvement in caring and their participation in the labour market has increased. She estimates that one in seven of those in the labour market have some involvement in caring. Clearly this is likely to increase in the future and, as such, employers may have to acknowledge this aspect of their employees lives.

The prevalence of caring among those defined as unemployed was 14% for men, 11% for non-married women and 20% for married women. Taking the case of men as an example, the prevalence of caring was highest among those defined as unemployed (14%) as compared with full-time (11%) and part-time employees (12%). It would be easy to draw the conclusion that caring 'causes' men to be unemployed. However it could also be that they have become carers because they are unemployed. This serves to reinforce the complexity of trying to determine the impact caring has upon carers lives.

Hancock and Jarvis (1994) have attempted to quantify the impact of caring by drawing a careful comparison between non-carers and ex-carers using secondary analysis of the OPCS survey of retirement and retirement plans. Among the sample of 3500 people, aged 55–69 years, and their partners they identified a sample of 390 male and 713 ex-carers (the characteristics of this group have been profiled in the section on becoming an ex-carer). Table 6.12 shows that 9% of ex-carers had changed their retirement plans because of their caring role and that, overall, 14% of men and 26% of women reported that caring had effected their employment (becoming unemployed, taking a lower paid job, difficulty getting a job or losing pay). Clearly this group of ex-carers perceived that their caring role had adversely effected their labour market participation. However the survey does not indicate whether this was a source of dissatisfaction to ex-carers.

Table 6.12 Effects of caring upon retirement plans and employment: past carers (%)[a]

	Male	Female
Effected retirement plans	7	10
Lost job and became unemployed because of caring	4	15
Took lower paid job because of caring	2	3
Had difficulty getting a job because of caring	3	4
Lost pay because of caring	10	11
At least one effect on employment	14	26

[a]Derived from: Hancock and Jarvis, 1994, Tables 5 and 6

How helpful are employers to the needs of employees who are also carers? In the 1996 CNA survey, 40% of carers who were employed reported that their employers were helpful to them in their role as carer. The most common form of employer support were 'flexible working hours' and 'a caring supportive attitude'.

It is not surprising that fulfilling the dual role of carer and employee results in problems for the carer. Laczko and Phillipson (1991) report that, according to the CNA, 88% of women employee carers and 44% of males, reported stress through fulfilling both these roles simultaneously. Laczko and Phillipson (1991, p. 41) report one carer as stating '... my work suffers due to lack of concentration when worried (about dependent). This in turn leads me to make mistakes which I worry about, firstly for inconvenience caused to customers/colleagues and secondly, for jeopardizing my chances of promotion/upgrading'. While also documenting the negative employment consequences of being a carer (time lost from work, reduced work performance, rearranging schedules and lost opportunities), Phillips (1994) observes that employment has beneficial aspects. These include: having a break from caring; opportunities for social interaction; an improved self esteem; as well as the material rewards. Although Laczko and Phillipson (1991) identify a need for employers to recognize the caring role undertaken by many employees, there has been little development of 'carer-friendly' employment practices.

Financial circumstances

The fulfilling of caring responsibilities may have an impact both when the carer is actively participating in the provision of care and may continue when they have discharged their caring responsibilities. Again, specifying precisely the effect of caring upon the financial circumstances of the carer is problematic because of some of the methodological issues noted above. Overall, carers appear to have a lower income than non-carers; they are less likely to be working, may work shorter hours and may receive lower rates of pay (Parker and Lawton, 1994; Joshi, 1995; Baldwin, 1995).

Evandrou (1991) reviewed the financial circumstances of different types of carer. This analysis revealed that 20% of female carers and 17% of male carers were in the bottom fifth of the income distribution, and 19% and 24% respectively were in the top fifth (for non-carers the percentages were 18% and 23%). However, when the data are analyzed by whether the carer lived with their dependent and the intensity of the caring relationship there was a different pattern. Of co-resident carers, 25% were in the bottom quintile; for extra-resident carers the percentages were 16% and 26% respectively. Sole carers (22%) are more likely to be in the bottom quintile than joint (11%) and peripheral (18%) and female sole carers were more likely to be in the bottom quintile than male carers (23% and 20% respectively). The advantaged position of employed carers compared with the economically inactive is revealed as 5% of this group are in the bottom quintile as compared with 32% of the inactive.

In summary, carers as a group experience lower income overall than non-carers. However when dealing with carers as a whole the difference is not especially great. However, when we subdivide the carer population into its district elements, we find that particular groups of carers are particularly disadvantaged. Female carers with sole responsibility for a co-resident dependent are the most financial disadvantaged group of carers.

Of those included in the 1992 CNA survey, 47% reported that they had experienced financial difficulties since becoming a carer (although of course we do not know that this is directly attributable to them undertaking a caring role). Financial problems were most likely to be reported by 'young' carers (i.e. those aged 35–64 years) as opposed to carers aged 65 years and over (61% and 31% respectively). However, it is difficult to determine if this represents a 'true' difference in the financial circumstances of individuals or differences in their expectations. When asked in this survey what single change would improve their quality of life, 20% carers responded 'more money' – both in terms of better benefits and in terms of what it could buy.

Although, in overall terms, the financial circumstances of current and ex-carers appear only marginally different from the general population this finding conceals several important facts. It is those carers with the highest levels of commitment, sole carers looking after a co-resident dependent who are the most financially disadvantaged. The majority of this group are women. Furthermore, although the income of carers and non-carers may show little marked divergence we do not know about the 'extra' costs incurred in looking after a disabled person. From this we may speculate that although income may vary little, expenditure is likely to be proportionately higher for those caring for a disabled relative. Hence it is likely that the above analysis under-estimates the financial costs of caring. Clearly to establish, rigorously, the financial and employment effects resulting from the provision of informal care longitudinal type studies are needed.

Health

We noted earlier that a significant number of carers are in the older age groups. From this we might speculate that a considerable number of carers may themselves experience health problems (some of which may be directly or indirectly associated with or exacerbated by their caring responsibilities). Evandrou (1991) reports that fewer carers described their health in the previous year as 'good' compared with the general population (58% and 63% respectively) and more described it as fairly good (29% and 25% respectively).

The 1992 CNA survey reported that 65% of carers reported that their health had been adversely affected by their caring responsibilities. Of those reporting health problems four main types were identified:

- 28% reported physical effects such as back strain e.g. 'pulled muscles give me terrible pain';
- 30% reported mental problems e.g. 'I'm depressed';
- 24% reported tiredness e.g. 'that totally shattered feeling of tiredness – I've not had an unbroken night's sleep for 10 years';
- 14% cited stress as a result of their caring role. High rates of stress among carers have been consistently reported (Nolan et al., 1990).

This survey also highlights the very low expectations of this group of individuals. 40% of the respondents answered that caring had not affected their health, half of these then wrote comments indicating that in fact they had health problems such as '… I have exhaustion, anxiety, depression and sometimes insomnia' and 'nothing really, just blood pressure caused by sleepless nights and worry' (CNA, 1992, p. 38). Clearly, carers, because of their age profile, are likely to be experiencing health problems which are exacerbated by fulfilling their caring role. However, we clearly need further work to try to tease out the adverse health effects resulting from caring and then to develop effective interventions which will alleviate these.

Given the high prevalence of health problems among carers, it is disturbing that 9% report that in the event of an accident no-one would know they were a carer (CNA,1996). Furthermore, 61% report that they had not thought about who would look after them if they could not manage because of illness, age or disability (this compares with 59% for the general population) (CNA, 1996).

Getting a break from caring

How often do carers manage to get a break from caring? According to the CNA (1992), 32% of carers did not get a regular break from their caring responsibility. This is reinforced by data from the 1985 GHS (Green, 1988) which reported that

52% of all carers had not had a two day break since becoming a carer. Co-resident carers were less likely to have had a two day break than extra-resident carers (57% and 35% respectively) (Evandrou, 1991). Arranging to have a break from caring was thought to be problematic. Of carers, where commitment consisted of a minimum of 20 hours a week, 44% thought that no-one else could look after the dependent if they wanted a two day break (49% of co-resident carers and 26% for extra-resident carers) and of the rest 34% thought that it was not difficult to arrange (again more of a problem for co-resident as compared with extra-resident carers – 29% and 51% respectively). Consequently, it is clearly difficult for carers to get a break or to organize spontaneous outings – careful planning is clearly required.

A NETWORK OF CARE?

We noted earlier that a substantial number of carers were solely responsible for the care of their dependents. In this section we explore the involvement of a caring network in the care of dependent people in the community. Overall, 23% of carers had sole responsibility for the care of their dependent. 30% reported that, although they received help, they spent more time than anyone else in caring for the dependent person, while 11% shared the main responsibility with someone else (Green, 1988). A much higher percentage of co-resident carers were sole carers (42%) compared with extra-resident carers (15%) (Green, 1988), and women were most likely to be sole carers than men (59% and 45% respectively). It is among co-resident carers looking after a spouse that we find the highest percentage of carers reporting that no-one else helped look after their dependent. Overall 70% of carers looking after a spouse reported that no-one else was involved (Green, 1988). This was greatest among women (77%) as compared with men (62%). Where people were caring for a parent then the percentage of lone carers was less marked. Overall 32% of co-resident carers looking after a parent (in law) were sole carers (25% of men and 36% of women) and 24% of extra-resident carers (12% of men and 31% of women). From this we can conclude that most of those caring for an elderly spouse do so largely unsupported by the wider community. This is less true for those caring for parents where the percentage of sole carers, though important, was lower. Finally these data suggest that women are more likely to be sole carers than men.

This isolation of carers and the lack of support they receive is reinforced by surveys conducted by the CNA. The 1996 survey indicated that almost half of all their carers (45%) did not receive any help with their dependent. Similarly their 1992 survey indicated that 33% of carers did not receive any support or help with their caring responsibilities. Where support was being received this came from the informal network of family rather than formal services (CNA, 1992). That the family is the first source of help is reinforced by the 1996 CNA survey. Respondents in this survey reported that if they wanted help with their caring responsibilities they would turn to their family (reported by 56%) rather than friends/neighbours (11%), GP (8%) or social services (20%).

Carers and formal services

If there is little involvement of other family, friends or neighbours in the provision of informal care in the community how involved are statutory and voluntary services. Are services from the formal sector involved in supplementing the work of informal carers? Limited data are available from the 1985 GHS survey (Green, 1988). This asked if dependents received regular (i.e. at least monthly) visits from a variety of health and social care agencies. Table 6.13 shows that only one fifth of carers were in regular contact with their GP and only 15% with a community/district nurse. Levels of service support are low for co-resident and extra-resident dependents indicating that services are received by only a minority of dependents. Rather than a network of informal carers being supported by statutory and voluntary services, it appears that most of those caring for an elderly person are left to do so on their own with only very minimal support from the formal sector. Despite the low levels of support carers appear to receive from statutory services they do report that they are satisfied with this (Allen *et al.*, 1992). However this may just reflect their low level expectations or a realization that there is little chance of more help.

Table 6.13 Regular receipt of services by carers: Great Britain, 1985[a]

| | Carers receiving services (%) | | |
	Co-resident carer	Extra-resident carer	All carers
District/community nurse	13	26	22
Health visitor	14	16	15
Social worker	5	6	6
Home help	3	7	7
Meals on wheels	1	10	7

[a]Derived from: Green, 1988, Table 5.8

It is too early to determine with any certainty the effect the implementation of the community changes has had upon carers. Warner (1994) in his survey of CNA members reports that 79% thought that the implementation of the the act had made no difference to the services they received. This study like many others highlighted carers key concerns with services:

- the perceived unreliability of services provided;
- difficulty with access to weekend services;
- difficulties in getting a break from caring (this ranged from regular weekly respite to longer breaks).

When asked what services they would like, the carers surveyed by Warner (1994) were very modest in their requests. Indeed he observes that in the focus groups, run as part of this project, carers were very loath to come up with 'a shopping list' of demands. The main request from the carers were for respite care. This ranged from home sitting for a few regular hours a week to regular day-care or an annual holiday break. Allen *et al.* (1992b), among others, also indicate that 70% of carers wanted more help and that the service most wanted was respite care. Support groups, where carers could meet other carers, were also seen as valuable in Warner's study. However this later type of service may not be so appealing to those carers who do not already belong to an organization. For example Allen *et al.* (1992b) report that 99% of those who had not been to a carers group did not want to go and felt that they were peripheral to their needs. Reliable high quality professional services were what the carers in this study wanted.

Who should help carers?

According to the members of the CNA three-quarters wanted more help and support and 69% thought it should come from the statutory sector rather than family or friends (CNA,1992). The main people who carers felt should give more help were family doctors (40%), respite services (38%) and social workers (32%).

Carers have fairly modest demands for help. In the 1992 CNA respondents were asked what single thing would improve their quality of life. The responses to this question fell into four main categories:

- 38% thought that the most important single improvement would be increased availability of respite care e.g. 'much more respite care. I spent 13 years without even one day's rest' and 'a complete break twice a year – say two weeks total – would be great'.
- 20% reported the need for more money e.g. 'if I could buy in help I would get the same person at a regular time to suit me – not the social services people who come in at their convenience, nice though they are'.
- 18% wanted practical help or adaptations in the home e.g. 'I'd love to give him a proper bath but I need a helper' or 'a walk-in shower would change our lives'.
- 14% felt they would be helped by more recognition and understanding of their problems by either their family or society e.g. 'if only the rest of the family would offer' or 'we need more acceptance of dementia so that people sympathize and then we could have action'.

CONCLUSION

In this chapter we have seen that the term 'carer' which implies, like many other social categories, a single homogeneous social group with a unique set of needs and circumstances is, in fact, a group composed of several different types of carers who will have differing needs and expectations of support from the formal sector. Initially research concerned with carers and caring sprang from the feminist research tradition. This obscured the fact that a significant number of carers are men. We can identify two distinct types of carers; spouses and siblings. Where the spouse is caring for the other marriage partner then the carer may be either male or female. However when the carer is a child caring for a parent (or parent in law) then the carer is most likely to be a daughter. These two different types of caring relationships develop for different reasons but are embedded in the complex web of family relationships. When considering the issues of informal care provision we need to specify the type of caring relationship (e.g. spouse, parent, etc.) and the context within which it is taking place (e.g. co-resident carer or extra-resident carer) and then provide the appropriate interventions. One problem is that so few interventions with carers have been evaluated. However it seems of little doubt that the provision of regular respite care would greatly improve the quality of life for carers. Overall we can conclude that there is little evidence that care for older people (and probably other client groups as well) is provided by a network of support provided by both informal and formal services working together. Rather, care is provided by a lone carer, usually a close family member, with very minimal state help. In the final chapter (Chapter 8) we will look at changes in the provision of family care over time and consider how the provision of informal care may change in future decades.

7

Long-stay care for older people

INTRODUCTION

The growth in state social security expenditure on private residential and nursing home care was the prime force in setting up the review of community care provision which subsequently resulted in the 1991 NHS and Community Care Act (Chapter 1). In this context long-stay care is care provided within an institutional environment and in which people are expected to remain for the remainder of their lives. In this chapter we will look more closely at the provision of long-stay (or continuing) care for older people and consider some of the key policy issues.

THE PROVISION OF LONG-STAY CARE

We can classify the different types of long-stay care provision for older people (or indeed other age groups) in two main ways; by the type of provider or the type of care being provided.

The providers of long stay care

There are three main providers of long-stay care; state services (provided either by the local authority or the NHS), the private sector and the voluntary sector.

Type of care provision

There are two main types of long-stay care; residential care and nursing/continuing NHS care. In the minds of policy makers at least there is a classification of older people into two distinct groups; those who need residential care and those who need nursing care. The origins of this dichotomy lie with the creation of the post-1945 welfare state and these are briefly discussed. As we shall see there are difficulties in deciding at what level of dependency each sector should take responsibility. However this difference is not one of mere semantics. There are important implications for older people and their families. Local authority provision has always expected that residents would contribute towards their care (if they were able) while NHS provided care is free at the point of consumption.

The origin of residential care

Residential care provision was, until recently, largely provided by local authority social service departments. This type of care originated with the 1948 National Assistance Act. Under the terms of this act local authorities were obliged to 'provide residential accommodation for all persons who because of age, infirmity or other reasons are in need of care and attention which is not otherwise available to them'. As this requirement was included in part three of the act these types of residential home became colloquially known as part three homes. Such care was seen as being locally available in modern purpose build homes, rather than in the old workhouses. However the austerity of post-war Britain meant that many of the intended homes were never built and the old workhouses continued to provide much of the residential care for older people. It was this type of provision about which Townsend was so scathing, referring to it as 'The Last Refuge' (Townsend, 1964).

The phrasing of the obligation is clearly open to interpretation in two different ways; what constitutes being 'in need' and what types of care and services should be provided to respond to the needs. This ambiguity in the original framing legislation means that there are no agreed criteria as to who needs this type of care and of what the pattern of care provided should consist. However we may speculate that the spirit of the legislation was such that it is doubtful that the architects of the act intended it for the immobile, incontinent or the demented. It is likely that such institutions were seen as providing a supported living environment for the physically frail as distinct from a hospital or nursing home where the 'sick' older person would receive care.

Some indication of the type of client the new 'part three' homes were aimed at may be gathered from the following quotations (Means and Smith, 1985, p. 181). Amulree, the geriatrician saw such homes as being for the able bodied as 'most of the residents will be able to keep their own rooms clean and tidy and may even be able to help with some of the general work of the household and the grounds'. Similarly, a deputy secretary at the DoH stated 'in the early days we thought old persons' homes were for active old people whose over-riding need was for accommodation both comfortable and suitable'. However soon after the creation of 'part three' homes the principle of residential care available to all relatively active older people was abandoned because of the shortages of care and the level of demand.

The provision of long-term health care

Long-stay care for those with medical or nursing care needs has, from 1948 until very recently, been provided mainly by the NHS. The provision of such care originates with the pre-1948 pattern of health care provision when the 'chronic sick' most of whom were elderly) were clustered in the Public Assistance Institutions. When these institutions were integrated into the NHS the health service took over responsibility for the care of the chronic, as well as acutely sick, and for rehabilitation. It is only fairly recently that the private sector has become a major provider of long-term nursing care for those who, while they do not need acute medical interventions, have a much higher level of dependency than would be deemed appropriate for residential care. We will look at the development of the nursing home sector later in this chapter.

Differentiating between residential and hospital care

In the organization of long-term care for older people there is an explicit assumption that it is possible to distinguish the frail (in need of residential care) from the sick (who would be most appropriately dealt with in a hospital/nursing home setting). However since the passing of the welfare state legislation in the immediate post-war period there have been continuing debates about the boundaries between these two sectors. The debate about what constitutes 'health care' and what properly constitutes the domain of 'social care' is not, therefore, a new one. Rather it represents the continuation of a longstanding tension between these two different types of care and the providers of such care.

Almost 10 years after the introduction of the National Assistance Act, guidance was issued by central government as to the type of older person who should be the recipient of residential care and those who should be the responsibility of health authorities. These are described below. However two points should be noted. First, it was accepted that interpretation of the guidance would be made locally. Second, and perhaps most importantly, the criteria were issued as guidance and therefore have no statutory power. These criteria did not convey the 'right' to care for anyone falling within the circumstances identified. The problems of distinguishing the boundaries between these various types of care is still current as is the definition of what older people may expect or be entitled to when they need care on an ongoing basis.

Who needs residential care?

Local authorities were advised in 1957 (circular 14/57) that they were responsible for providing residential care for 'the active older person' (MoH, 1957) as well as:

the care of residents during a minor (implied acute self-limiting) illness which may require a period (unspecified) in bed;
the care of the infirm who may need help with dressing, using the toilet, who may be unable to cope with stairs and who may have to spend part of the day in bed;
those bedbound residents with terminal illness and who would not benefit from further medical intervention.

It was clearly not regarded as the province of the local authority to provide extensive and continuing nursing care. However there are obviously problems in interpreting this guidance. Care in a residential home for terminally ill residents wa acceptable if they were expected to die within weeks. However death is not always so predictable. It was not seen as desirable to develop 'infirmary' wards as annexes to residential homes to care for residents as their health care needs became greater. Rather, such older people were seen as having to move to the hospital sector if they had major health care needs. However Means and Smith (1985) speculate that hospitals remained very reluctant to admit residents from residential homes while the latter rarely relished the prospect of nursing care for frail residents. These authors observed that hospitals and homes developed 'local bargaining' and would 'swop' residents between sectors (e.g. a hospital would admit a sick person from a residential home if they would accept a patient from a geriatric ward in return). In all this the needs and wishes of the older person were subjugated to the needs of the institutions involved.

Circular 18/65 on *The Care of the Elderly in Hospitals and Residential Homes* (MoH, 1965) was an attempt to re-emphasize the boundary lines. This restated that the residential sector was to care for:

- elderly people, who after careful assessment of their medical and social needs are unable to maintain themselves in their own homes, even with full support including;
- people so incapacitated that they need help with dressing, toileting and meals but who are able to get about with a walking aid or with some help by wheel chair;
- people using appliances that they can manage themselves or without nursing assistance;
- people with temporary or continuing confusion of the mind but who do not need psychiatric nursing care.

The circular also stated that residents who fell ill should be cared for in the home if the illness would normally be managed at home, patients with terminal disease should not be transferred to hospital unless medically indicated and incontinent residents should also remain in the home. The definition of who residential care was aimed at had developed from the initial notion that it was for the 'able bodied' but 'frail' older person. The boundary issue has never really been resolved and surveys have consistently shown an overlap between hospitals and residential homes in the levels of dependency of older patients for whom they are caring.

Who needs hospital care?

The hospital authorities were seen as being providers of care for the acutely sick older person and those needing active treatment such as rehabilitation. In addition they were, as stated in circular HM(57)86 (MoH, 1957), seen as being responsible for:

- the care of the chronic bedfast who, while not needing medical treatment or intervention, required nursing care over a prolonged period;

- the 'convalescent' care of the elderly sick who have finished their treatment but are not yet ready for discharge;
- the confused or disturbed patient who, because of his/her condition, is not fit to live in the community or a residential home.

The circular indicated that hospital authorities did not have to give all the medical or nursing care needed by an old person, nor did they have to admit all those who required nursing care. Hence there has always been rationing of access to medical care for older people. This is not simply a new phenomena associated with the 1991 changes to the health services, especially the creation of the internal market.

Two main policy points which are still relevant are highlighted by this guidance. First, this guidance is full of ambiguities of interpretation (Means and Smith, 1985). Although further guidance has been issued (e.g. in circular 18/65: the care of the elderly in hospitals and residential homes) the boundary debate about who provides what type of care for which type of older person persists. The problem of 'the partly sick partly well older person' still challenges the system which seeks to dichotomize these two states. Second, it did not confirm any rights or entitlements to care for older people and neither has any subsequent policy document. What older people can expect from the welfare state in terms of long-stay care (or indeed any other form of support) has varied over time and also varies locally. Equity of access of provision was never a guiding principle for social services even if it was in theory at least a cornerstone of the NHS.

The implementation of the NHSCCA has again served to draw attention to the boundary between health and social care. Furthermore the financial differences between sectors have also been highlighted as the act has come into force. Those who are seeking public support for entry into nursing or residential homes must pay towards their care if they have assets above a specified level; recipients of NHS care (either long-term or domiciliary nursing) are not expected to contribute. This anomaly has been identified by the House Of Commons Select Committee on Health (1996) who recommended that the NHS should accept financial responsibility for the nursing component of long-stay care.

Resulting from the debate about the responsibilities of the NHS, and the development of concerns that the NHS was withdrawing from rehabilitation and long-term care to concentrate upon acute work, guidance as to the responsibilities of the NHS for meeting continuing health care needs was issued (HSG (95)8) (DoH, 1995a). This states that the NHS is responsible for arranging and funding the following services;

- specialist medical and nursing assessment;
- rehabilitation and recovery;
- palliative health care;
- continuing inpatient care under specialist supervision in hospital or nursing home;
- respite health care;
- specialist health care support for people in nursing and residential homes or in the community;

- community health services for people at home or in residential care homes;
- primary health care;
- specialist transport services.

However the guidance states that such services must be made available within existing resources, that these services must compete with other priorities and that the balance of services is likely to vary between areas. It is this guidance which states that patients do not have the right to an indefinite NHS bed but that they can refuse to be discharged to a nursing or residential home. In such cases they would be discharged home with a package of care within the options and resources available.

THE REGULATION OF LONG-STAY CARE

The provision of long-stay care is subject to both registration and inspection procedures. Since April 1991, local authorities have been required to have 'inspection units'. The rationale for this being that inspection is one way in which the quality of the services provided can be ensured. Inspection units, as well as reviewing residential care which they are required to do, may also review domiciliary or day-care services. However they have no statutory obligations to undertake such activities.

Local authorities are responsible for the registration of private and voluntary homes within their area and for the inspection of all residential homes (including those provided by the local authority). Nursing homes are registered and inspected by the district health authority under separate legislation. Some homes are 'dual registered' as both residential and nursing homes which means that two separate agencies are involved in registration and inspection. Hence the system for the regulation and inspection of long-term care perpetuates the distinction between the frail and the sick. Furthermore there is no system for the registration and inspection of long-term care provided by the NHS.

ELIGIBILITY FOR LONG-STAY CARE

Under the new community care changes, entry to long-stay residential and nursing home care at the public expense is through the assessment of individual need. So, while there is a uniform system for entering residential and nursing home care, the position regarding access to long-stay geriatric beds remains ambiguous and clearly remains under the control of the medical profession (largely geriatricians). How are individuals' needs for admission to such types of care assessed. While all agencies have procedures the legislative requirements are being implemented in a myriad of different ways. It seems that there is no single model of how this process operates.

There is a further complication. Services provided by the local authority have always been subject to means-testing. Through the charging system, users have always made contributions, if they are judged able, to the cost of services provided. This has always been the case for local authority part three care. However long-stay care services provided by the NHS have always been free at the point of consumption. So, as well as differences in the means of accessing services there are also differences in the expectations about older people's contribution to such services. The new system has served to highlight and accentuate these differences but as yet they have not been resolved. However one result of the impact of the community care changes has been to turn the neglected issue of long-term care provision into a topic which is now on the political agenda (House of Commons Select Committee on Health, 1996).

Under the new arrangements health authorities, in collaboration with local authorities and GPs had to produce local policies and eligibility criteria for continuing health care. These should compliment those criteria produced by local authorities for residential care to avoid people falling between the two policies (the boundary between the frail and the sick). The guidance issued by central government in this area relates to the items the local policies must address e.g. assessment of need, monitoring and evaluation and the availability of written documentation. However central guidance does not spell out what types of problems are the responsibility of the NHS and what fall within the jurisdiction of the residential care services. It is expected that these decisions will be made locally. This introduction of 'local variation' into the provision of NHS services does not fit easily with the founding principles of the NHS which was of equity of access to health care services. We will explore some of the problems in the area of continuing care and its relationship with the acute hospital sector in a later section.

Eligibility for NHS care : the ACC/AMA survey

The survey conducted by the Association of County Councils/Association of Metropolitan Authorities (ACA/AMA, 1995) provides some clues as to how individual local authorities are defining those groups seen as eligible for residential/nursing home care. They sent 10 case profiles to 74 local authorities and asked them to describe which services would be given. We have already used examples from this survey (Chapter 5) when looking at the contribution of formal domiciliary based services. Here we use the profiles relating to individuals at the boundary for entry into different types of long-term care. For each case the 'real' outcome of their referral is also reported (Table 7.1). Case 1 was selected by the survey team as it is a typical example of the changing boundaries between health and social care and typifies the dilemmas experienced by local authorities when receiving referrals from acute hospitals. This was a man with an inoperable brain tumour of uncertain prognosis who was in pain and needed constant nursing care. Only 14% of responders thought that this case was the responsibility of the NHS while 86% would have accepted responsibility for his nursing home care; one consequence of which would be that there would be a charge to this person for his

care. With regard to this case the report notes problems in reaching local agreements on the division of responsibilities. They comment that even when formal
local agreements did exist doubts were expressed that the NHS would provide services. Furthermore when agreements existed, comments were made about the
interpretation of eligibility criteria. The real outcome for this case was that the
patient was referred for hospice care but no place was available. This case would
appear to be firmly within the responsibilities of the NHS as laid out in circular
HSG (95) 8 LAC (95)5 (DoH, 1995a) described above as this patient was clearly
in need of palliative care. This would appear to be an example of where the NHS
is trying to redefine health needs as social care needs and is something that social
services maintain is putting their budgets under stress. They have been funded on
the basis of accepting responsibility for providing community care needs not for
the redefinition of the boundary between health and social care.

Eligibility for residential/nursing home care

How are local authorities deciding who needs nursing home care, who needs residential care and who can be cared for at home? Again the ACC/AMA survey provides some insights into the thinking of the lead agencies. The case profiles shown
in Tables 7.1 and 5.18 illustrate a range of different circumstances. Cases 3, 4, 5 and
8 were thought to have needs which could be most appropriately met by residential
or nursing home care by a significant percentage of the responding local authorities.
   These cases all highlight different dimensions of the boundary between domiciliary and long-stay care and the types of service allocation decisions with which local
authorities have to deal. Case 3 highlights the situation where an informal carer is
undertaking a significant caring role. We have already noted the contribution of informal carers but for how long can local authorities expect them to act as a resource?
   One of the issues which has to be confronted by local authorities is how long
intensive community care packages can be sustained. When a client is clearly
deteriorating how long can they be sustained. At what point should the move to
residential care be made? These questions cannot be answered by the survey but
this case profile (number 3) does highlight the complexity of the issues being confronted by local authorities and the variation in the way they respond to them. One
aspect of this is that the expense of providing intensive home care packages can
exceed the cost of residential or nursing home provision. So, at some point it is
cheaper to provide communal care rather than care at home.
   Case 5 highlights issues around hospital discharge, an area which we have previously seen has been problematic almost from the creation of the NHS. Interestingly, although this person had dementia, virtually no responding authorities
thought him the responsibility of the NHS. The real outcome for this patient was
that his wife did not want him discharged from hospital but would not sanction
nursing home care. Although there is a procedure for patients to challenge the
decision to discharge them from NHS care, they do not have the right to remain in
hospital care indefinitely.

Table 7.1 Case profiles of clients 'at risk' of entry into residential/nursing home care[a]

Case number	Profiles
1	A 71–year-old male living with his wife. Son lives away. Paralysis on right side and loss of vision due to inoperable brain tumour discovered after an emergency hospital admission. Uncertain prognosis. Needs constant attention for pain and constant nursing care. Family considers he needs specialist care. This case illustrates the changing boundary between health and social care. This case should have been an NHS responsibility as palliative care is an NHS responsibility for those with a likely short time to live. Actual outcome: referred for hospice care but no vacancies. Stayed in hospital as family resisted all attempts to discharge him to a nursing home or home care as they did not think he was fit to leave hospital. Died within four weeks of emergency admission.
3	An 81-year-old man living alone. Visited regularly by niece who also cares for her mother. Discharged after a lengthy hospital stay. Is incontinent and in the early stages of dementia. This illustrates a case where there is a carer, and raises the questions of what support she should receive. Actual outcome: refused home care. Offered limited help with incontinence
4	A 90-year-old widow is living alone, but is visited regularly by son. Has heart disease and circulatory problems. Numerous hospital admissions. Very frail. Walks with a zimmer. GP and district nurse visit regularly. Needs help with personal care, getting up and dressing. This case illustrates a person on the verge of admission to residential care, and raises the issue of how long a clearly deteriorating situation can continue. When is the 'right' time to move into care? Actual outcome: discharged from hospital with daily home care. Fell within seven days of discharge. Readmitted to hospital. Discharged to residential care and died nine days after admission.
5	A 76-year-old man lives with wife. No other support. Has Alzheimer's disease. Ready for hospital discharge. Wife has cared for six years and is exhausted. He needs help to feed, dress, bathe and get in/out of bed. Is doubly incontinent. This illustrates a long term care situation where intensive personal and social care provided by an informal carer. Actual outcome: referred for a nursing home place but wife resisted discharge from hospital.
8	A 72-year-old widow who lives alone. No family support. Exhibits agitated, violent and bizarre behaviour. Wanders. Needs help to dress and feed and toilet. This is a person with extensive social and personal needs. Actual outcome: placed in a nursing home.

Derived from: ACA/AMA, 1995

Case 8, which again highlights the issue of dementia, illustrates the very extensive social and personal care needs such clients can present. Again a minority of responding local authorities considered this client should be cared for by the NHS. The majority would offer nursing home care to this type of client and this was where this client was placed.

These case profiles raise a number of important issues with regard to the provision of continuing care services. Given the level of need, it would have seemed reasonable to expect that some of situations would have been seen as the responsibility of the NHS. These data seem to imply that there is little expectation from the local authorities surveyed that the NHS will continue to offer long-stay services. These profiles resulted in some clear uniformity of decision-making by authorities. Cases 7 and 10 (Chapter 5) were seen as appropriate for home care. Cases 1, 5 and 8 (Table 7.2) were largely seen as falling within the domain of nursing home care. In contrast to the apparently clear and consistent allocation of home or nursing home care the role of residential care was not clear and showed overlap with the other two types of care. The ambiguity regarding the role of residential care which has existed almost since its creation continues. The 'place in the market' of this type of care still remains ill-defined.

Table 7.2 Outcome for case profiles[a]

Case	Met eligibility criteria (%)	Offered nursing home (%)	Offered residential (%)
1	86	79	0
3	98	5	21
4	100	6	24
5	99	60	13
8	98	31	42

[a]Derived from: ACA/AMA, 1995, Tables 3 and 9

THE SUPPLY OF LONG-STAY CARE

How much long-stay care is available for older people? What is the balance between the different sectors and types of provision? Answering these apparently simple questions can be very problematic because of the way that data collection concerning provision has changed over time. For some sectors data are routinely collected (e.g. the number of residential home places) while for others, such as the number of long-stay NHS beds, it is not. Our analysis is further constrained because of the limitation imposed by the way that official data is presented (e.g. not differentiating between the provision given to different client groups such as the younger disabled and older people).

We may consider the availability of long-stay care in four distinct ways:

• the number of institutions providing care;

- the number of places available;
- the number and types of residents;
- the number of publicly supported residents (i.e. who pays for the care provided).

In the discussion of levels of provision we will confine our attention to the first three aspects of the availability of long-term care and will consider them within each of the main provider groups (private, voluntary and statutory) and types of provision (i.e. nursing home, residential and NHS). We shall return to the issue of who pays for long-stay care in a later section.

Residential care provision

As of March 31st 1995 there were 16 320 staffed residential homes in England (excluding 'small' homes with four or less residents). These homes provided 329 200 places and had 288 600 residents. There were a further 5500 small homes with 10 300 residents (DoH, 1996).

The distribution of residential care by the different types of provider (e.g. public, private and voluntary) is shown in Table 7.3 This reveals that the private sector is now responsible for 62.6% of residential homes, 56.9% of residential care places and cares for 56% of residential care residents. It also shows the very marked decline of the local authority as a direct provider of residential care. However the role of the private sector as the main provider of residential care is fairly recent for it was not until 1989 that they reached this position. (DoH, 1996).

Table 7.3 Residential care in England, 1987–1995[a]

		Local authority	Private	Voluntary
Homes	1987	3410	7550	1560
	1995	2550	10 230	3540
Change (%)		-25.3	+35.4	+226
Places	1987	128 700	113 600	41 500
	1995	75 500	187 400	66 400
change (%)		-41.4	+64.9	+60.0
Residents	1987	114 000	93 700	34 600
	1995	66 500	161 700	60 400
Change (%)		-41.7	+72.5	+74.5

[a]Derived from: DoH, 1996, Table E

The data described above relate to all client groups in residential care. This includes the younger physically disabled, those with learning disabilities as well as older people. However, older people are the main consumers of residential care places occupying 81% of care places. If we confine our attention to older people, then in March 1995 there were 10 870 homes, offering 258 700 places and caring for 225 600 residents. Overall, 61% of older people in residential care are in privately run establishments and 55% of residents are aged 85 years or over. We will discuss the nature and characteristics of older people in residential care, and indeed other parts of the long-stay sector, later in this chapter.

Nursing home provision

The provision of nursing home care is the almost exclusive prerogative of the private sector, although there is some voluntary sector involvement. The potential of the NHS to provide long-stay care in nursing home settings has been evaluated (Clarke and Bowling, 1989) and indeed supported by the House of Commons Select Committee on Health (1996). However, there has been little enthusiasm among health care providers to develop such services.

Routine data do not indicate the number of nursing homes. The number of nursing home places in England in 1981 was estimated at 18 200 (House of Commons Select Committee on Health, 1996). This had increased to 109 000 by 1991; an increase of 90 800 places or 598% in a decade. As of 1994, it is estimated that the number of places had further increased to 148 500 (House of Commons Select Committee on Health, 1996). We may confidently speculate that the vast majority of nursing home residents are older people. The vast expansion of private nursing home and residential care arose because of changes in the way that means-tested benefits were paid to older people. At its most basic, people on low income could enter care, regardless of their 'need' as indicated by disability/dependence, and get their fees paid by the social security system. We will examine the financial consequences of this in a later section dealing with expenditure on long-stay care.

Hospital provision

Long-stay care for older people has traditionally been provided free of charge by the NHS. A distinction was usually drawn between those who were physically frail and those who were mentally frail. Information concerning the amount and type of long-stay beds provided by the NHS is not readily available. Although we know there has been a marked decline in the number of hospital beds. Tinker *et al.* (1994) report that the number of hospital beds in England decreased by more than a quarter between 1981 and 1991 (from 352 000 to 255 000). Beds dedicated to the specialty of geriatric medicine, for acute treatment, rehabilitation and long-stay care in the UK decreased from 67 628 in 1987/88 to 60 948 in 1991. However, it is not clear how many of the available beds were used for long-stay care and if the decreased availability of beds has occurred disproportionately in the long-stay sector. Taking a longer term view, Impallomeni and Star (1995) observe that 35% of geriatric beds in England (20 000 beds) were lost during the decade 1985–1994 and that most of these losses occurred in the long-stay sector. Further they note that psychogeriatric beds decreased by 29% (5000) during the period 1991–1994.

However, these data do not relate specifically to long-stay care beds. In 1980, Bosanquet and Gray (1989) estimated that there were 54 500 long-stay beds available in England. This represented about 23% of all long-stay places. These authors estimated that by 1985 the number of such places had decreased slightly to 54 100. Laing (1993) estimates that there are now 35 000 long-stay beds available in England and that this figure is continuing to decline.

The overall provision of long-stay care

Taking each of these sectors together, Table 7.4 suggests that there are 465 000 long-term care places. This indicates that the number of places has increased by 75% over the last decade. There has been a growth of 51.7% in residential care over the decade. So, although the rhetoric of the last decade has been towards the development of community (i.e. non-institutional) care, the reality has been a marked growth, in terms of absolute numbers, in long-stay provision.

Table 7.4 Long-stay care provision: England, 1981–1994[a]

Type of provision	Estimated places	
	1981	1994
NHS	54 500	35 000
Nursing home	18 200	148 500
Local authority	114 900	68 900
Voluntary residential	36 900	45 500
Private residential	39 300	164 200
Total	263 800	465 000
Rate per 100 aged 65+	3.7	5.7

[a]Derived from: House of Commons Select Committee on Health, 1996

Clearly, the number of older people has also increased over the period so any absolute increase in numbers could simply reflect this demographic shift. However, when expressed as a rate per 1000 population aged 65 years and over, it does seem that there has been a 'real' increase in long-term care places (from 3.5 places per 100 to 5.7). As we have already noted this expansion has taken place in the private sector provision rather than NHS or local authority provided services. However this relatively modest increase in the percentage of older people living in communal establishments is explained by the demographic change which took place over this period. Laing (1993) reports that the increase in the number of older people in long-stay care over the decade 1981–1992 was fairly modest. He applied age-specific rates of communal living for 1981 to the population of 1991 and estimated the number of people who would have been in care. He then compared this with the actual number. This revealed that there were 27% more people in care than would have been expected using 1981 rates. This increase is much less dramatic than the 65% increase in the number of absolute places available described above. Furthermore Laing's analysis assumes that there were no changes in morbidity during this decade.

There are major geographical variation in the availability of nursing and residential home care. Table 7.5 shows that there are major differences in the numbers of places between the counties and the urban areas, especially London. Access to residential home care is much less in the urban areas. These areas also have a much lower involvement of the private sector, possibly because suitable property is not available or is too expensive. However this table serves to emphasize that the types of services older people can expect to have access to will vary enormously depending upon which part of the country they live.

Table 7.5 Places in homes for older people by type of local authority: England, 1994[a]

	Places per 1000 aged 75+		Percentage residential places in independent sector
	Residential	Nursing	
Shire counties	82	77	48
Metro areas	69	67	50
Inner London	49	41	18
Outer London	50	67	19
England	75	73	45

[a]Derived from: DoH, 1996, Table 01

HOW MANY OLDER PEOPLE ARE IN LONG-STAY CARE?

It is difficult to give a precise statement as to the total number of older people who are resident in the different types of long-stay care. As we have already seen, routine sources provide only limited data about the residents of such accommodation. The best available information comes from the 1991 census. This revealed that 5% of those aged 60 years and over (101 100 men and 335 900 women) were resident in either long-stay hospital beds, residential homes or nursing homes (often referred to collectively as communal establishments) in Great Britain.

There is a very strong relationship between age, sex and the probability of living in a communal establishment in later life (Table 7.6). In numerical terms women are three times more likely to reside in such establishments as men. We may speculate that this reflects their greater susceptibility to chronic illness and the lack of others (namely a spouse) to care for them. While approximately 1% of those aged 60/65–74 years live in communal settings, this increases markedly for those aged 85 years and over (11% of men and 20% for women).

Table 7.6 also reinforces the importance of the role of the private sector. Of the 426 100 people aged 60/65 years and over living in communal establishments 65.9% were in private sector care (127 400 in private nursing homes, 153 400 in private residential homes and 93 700 in local authority homes). The number of people resident in NHS hospitals (either psychiatric or other) was much fewer at approximately 47 000.

Table 7.6 Population in medical and care establishment: Great Britain, 1991[a]

| | Male | | | Female | | |
	65–74	75–84	85+	60–74	75–84	85+
NHS hospitals	2.63	5.48	11.57	2.03	6.72	19.17
Private hospitals	0.2	0.41	1.0	0.18	0.52	1.55
LA homes	0.49	1.02	3.18	0.27	1.64	5.86
Nursing homes/private	2.71	11.75	44.92	2.78	20.20	77.75
Residential homes/private	3.16	12.05	53.16	3.17	23.98	100.30
Total	9.19	30.71	113.83	8.43	53.06	204.63

Rate per 1000

[a]Derived from: Jarvis *et al.*, 1996, Table A1

We may conclude that there has been some growth in the number of older people living in communal settings in England. Most of this increase is accounted for population ageing rather than vast increases in demand. Taking a longer term perspective, there has been a slight upward trend in the percentage of older people living in communal settings, from 4% in 1981 to 5% in 1991. However this increase is almost totally confined to the very old (i.e. those aged 85 years or over); from 19% in 1981 to 23% in 1991.

At a local level, Stern *et al.* (1993) have documented the changes in the availability of different types of long-stay care provision. They compared long-stay care provision for older people in Leicestershire between 1979 and 1990. They reported that in 1979 there were 4687 people aged 65 years and over resident in long-stay care; an overall rate of 4.2% compared with 4.7% in 1990 (a total of 6079 residents). So, although the survey enumerated an almost 30% increase in the number of residents this increase had only slightly outpaced the increase in the percentage of elderly people in the county. This mirrors the national trends described above. It also demonstrates the 'ageing' of the population being cared for by this sector; almost one half (44%) are now aged over 85 years compared with 35.2% in 1979.

The growth in importance of the private sector as a provider of long-stay care is echoed by the Leicestershire survey. In 1979, 83.6% of long-stay residents were accommodated by the public sector compared with 53.95% in 1990. However there are marked variations between local authorities in England (and within the other parts of the UK) in both the availability of long-stay care and the pattern of provision. For example a survey by the author of all long-stay care provision available in the London Borough of Kensington and Chelsea, undertaken in 1993, presents a different picture to that described in Leicestershire. Of the 1111 places enumerated, 66% were in the public sector. This illustrates that the growth of private sector care has not been equally distributed across the country but has been most prolific in non-metropolitan areas. Similarly, in Kensington and Chelsea there were, in 1993, 2.4% of those aged 65 years and over in long-stay care. This is less than half the national figure. Hence in some areas of the country the development of long-stay care provision has not kept pace with demographic change.

THE CHARACTERISTICS OF OLDER PEOPLE IN LONG-STAY CARE

What types of older people are being cared for by the long-term care sector and what degree of physical and mental frailty do such people exhibit? We saw earlier that, in the minds of policy makers at least, the residential care sector is supposed to be accommodating a much less frail population than nursing homes or long-stay NHS care. We would therefore expect that the disability and dependency profiles of these two types of care setting would be distinct and that these differences would also be reflected in the socio-demographic profile of residents.

The demographic profile of the long-stay care population

Women and the very old (i.e. those aged 85 years and over) are the most likely groups to be resident in long-stay care. This demographic profile is confirmed by both local (e.g. Stern *et al.*, 1993; Victor, 1991) and national (e.g. Darton and Wright, 1991) surveys of the residents of long-stay care. Within the Royal Borough of Kensington and Chelsea in London, approximately one-fifth of those in long-stay care were male and approximately half were aged 85 years or older. However, there is little difference in the age-sex composition of residents in the different forms of long stay care. Darton and Wright (1991) report the mean age of nursing home/residential care residents in their national survey as 83 years.

When we compare the ages of men and women in care some differences emerge. The average age of men in care is younger than that for women. Darton and Wright (1991) report that the average age of men in private nursing homes was 76 years compared with 84 years for women. It is probable that similar differences are observable in the other types of long-stay care. In the Kensington survey only a small minority of residents were still married; the majority were either single, divorced or widowed. This suggests that, among other factors, it is the lack of a caring network which is a factor indicative of entry into care.

Changes in the demographic profile over time

Has the socio-demographic profile of those resident in long-stay care changed? The Leicestershire survey provides some indication of the stability of the characteristics of older people in care. This study reveals that the population in long-stay care is itself ageing. In 1979, they reported that 22.4% of long-term care residents were aged 65–74 years and 35.2% were aged 85 years or over. By 1991 only 15.9% of residents were aged 65–74 years while 44.2% were aged 85 years and over. This illustrates that, in relative terms, the age profile of long-term care residents is increasing.

Levels of disability and dependency in long-stay care

Providing a definitive profile of the levels of disability, dependence and frailty of residents in long-stay care is problematic. Although there are a considerable number of studies of the physical and mental health status of these populations comparisons between studies are difficult because they have not all used the same assessment instruments. Each study has used a specific set of measurements tools not all of which are standardized instruments. However most tools cover similar areas such as mobility, continence, mental status, self-care. This enables some very crude comparisons to be made.

Table 7.7 Prevalence of different type of disability in long-stay care: a comparison of two studies

| | | Percentage having difficulties Type of care | | |
	NHS	Local authority	Private/ residential	Private/ nursing
Mobility (KC)[a]	78	79	57	87
Dressing (KC)	93	51	47	69
Darton and Wright[b]	-	30	32	56
Bathing (KC)	97	71	61	95
Darton and Wright	-	73	66	82
Incontinent (KC)	90	46	38	64
Darton and Wright	-	24	19	38
Dementia (KC)	64	61	49	59
Darton and Wright	-	59	48	63

[a]KC = Royal Borough of Kensington and Chelsea
[b]Darton and Wright, 1991, national sample of homes

Table 7.7 illustrates the very high prevalence of disability and dependency among this long-stay population as compared with the general population of older people. Although there are differences between studies, which reflects methodological differences, there are consistent patterns which may be observed. The first is the very dependent nature of this population; the majority have mobility problems, are unable to feed themselves, cannot dress themselves, suffer from incontinence and confusion. Second, there is evidence of differences in the prevalence of dependency between residential and NHS/nursing home care. As would be expected, the dependency levels are lower in residential care than NHS/nursing home care. However the population profile presented for the residential care sector does not conform to the 'frail but fit' ideal of residential care. Third, the extremely disabled nature of the population in NHS/nursing home care is striking. These data illustrate very high rates of immobility, dependency in self-care, incontinence and mental confusion. This should be borne in mind when we are considering the possibility of substituting community for institutional forms of care for this population.

Given the changing age-profile of the long-stay care population described earlier, it would be surprising if dependency levels had not increased. Stern *et al.* (1993) report that, when allowing for age and sex composition changes, the levels of disability in long-stay care residents increased between 1979 and 1991. It seems highly unlikely that this observation is specific to the study area of Leicestershire.

How long do residents remain in long-stay care?

To answer this question completely we would have to look at a cohort of admissions to long-stay care and then follow them up longitudinally. In the absence of such data, we have to compare the length of time people have been resident in care derived from cross-sectional studies. This is problematic because such studies over-emphasize the number of residents who have been resident for a considerable period of time. Given this caveat, Table 7.8 compares length of stay for residents in the different long-stay care settings and compares two studies (one from the Royal Borough of Kensington and Chelsea, and the second a national survey). Within both the NHS and nursing home sector the majority of residents were fairly recent arrivals; 50% of NHS patients and 40% of nursing home patients had been resident for under a year. Length of stay was longer in the residential sector with approximately a fifth of residents having been there for five years or more. Hence, while there is a fairly rapid turn-over of residents in these types of environments some people, especially in the residential sector, can spend a considerable period of time in care.

Table 7.8 Length of stay in long-stay care: a comparison of two studies

| | | Percentage length of stay Type of care | | |
	NHS	Local authority	Private/ residential	Private/ nursing
Under 1 year (KC)[a]	50	24	27	43
Darton and Wright[b]	-	31	44	41
1–3 years (KC)	28	32	41	27
Darton and Wright	-	33	39	37
3–5 years (KC)	14	15	11	15
Darton and Wright	-	16	10	14
5+ years (KC)	8	29	21	15
Darton and Wright	-	6	27	8

[a]KC = Royal Borough of Kensington and Chelsea
[b]Darton and Wright, 1991, national sample of homes

The average length of stay in private sector homes has been estimated at 2.5 years which suggests an average turnover of residents of 40% (Hamnet, 1995). If there are 470 000 nursing and residential home places then there could be 190 000 new entrants to care every year. Using a more conservative turnover rate of 25%, this still implies 125 000 new entrants annually. Consequently there are fairly extensive numbers of older people moving into care each year.

HOW DO PEOPLE ENTER LONG-STAY CARE?

How do older people end up being admitted to long-term care? What sort of circumstances result in this outcome? Remarkably little is known about how older people come to be admitted to long-term care and how the precipitating factors vary between the different sorts of long-stay care. This is because most of the research in this field has been of a cross-sectional nature and has been more concerned with determining the extent of 'mis-allocation' of residents between sectors than in looking at why people entered care in the first place.

Ideally, we need studies of a longitudinal design which follow people over time to try to determine how and why people end up being admitted to long-stay care. However, data from cross-sectional studies provide some clues as to the circumstances which might result in such an outcome.

One way to look at this is to examine the residential situation for older people prior to admission. In Kensington and Chelsea, a significant percentage of older people were admitted to long-stay care from hospital. This is especially true for those admitted to NHS/nursing home care. For example 31% of those ending up in an NHS long-stay ward were admitted from an acute ward. This compares with 19% and 10% for public residential homes and private residential homes respectively. In south London, it was reported that 90% of entrants to nursing homes were admitted from hospital (House of Commons Select Committee on Health, 1996). This highlights the importance of the relationship between hospitals and the long-stay sector. Delays in assessing older people for nursing care could adversely affect the way acute beds are used. This may encourage all concerned to speed up the nursing home admission process, however, although it may prevent (or reduce) the choice and participation of the older person.

The entry to residential care is most likely from the older person's own home. In the above study, over 50% of entrants to all forms of residential care came from their own home into care. A similar observation is reported by Allen *et al.* (1992b). This hints at different underlying factors precipitating entry into the two main types of care.

Why are older people admitted to care? For those within the NHS/nursing home sector the main precipitating factor, in Kensington and Chelsea, was an acute deterioration in their heath status (78%). For most of the people included in this category (85%), this was as a result of a major stroke which left the person severely disabled and unable to care for themselves. Hence entry into nursing care appears to be precipitated largely by a devastating change in the health status of the older person.

Entry into residential care may also result from changed/deteriorating health status. Allen *et al.* (1992b) report that 52% of admissions to residential care were due to this factor (45% in K and C). The importance of the caring network in maintaining older people in the community is also important. Both Allen *et al.* (1992b) and the K and C study identify the inability of carers or statutory services to cope with the level of disability presented by the older person as precipitating factors for entry into care. Again this hints at a change in the older person's disability to which carers, either formal or informal, could not respond. These responses should be interpreted in the light of the very severe levels of disability and dependency which characterize residents of long-stay care settings.

A percentage of entrants to care, especially private residential homes, 'choose' to go into care. Without interviewing the residents directly, it is difficult to interpret this. Was the choice a 'positive' one or was it because of the lack of a suitable alternative? These data, however, relate to those who had entered care before the implementation of the community care changes. Under the new arrangements older people will only be able to enter care, if they are seeking public support, if they are assessed as 'needing' care. This gives the impression that significant numbers of older people were entering residential care who did not 'need' such care. This thesis is not supported by the dependency profile of the population. Bradshaw and Gibbs (1988) report that, for admissions to residential care supported by the social security budget, only 7% failed to meet the eligibility criteria used for admissions to local authority part three homes. Furthermore, they report that only 17% of admissions could have been 'avoided' if additional domiciliary services such as day care or night sitting had been available.

Allen *et al.* (1992b) shed some light upon how older people enter residential care. Of their sample, 19% requested entry to care; for the remainder, entry into care was suggested by someone else (usually the carer or a professional health/social worker). This confirms Sinclair's (1988) observation that residential (and presumable nursing home care) is suggested by someone else. For the group of new entrants to care surveyed by Allen *et al.* (1992b) only 6% reported any alternative to residential care being discussed with them, and only 22% felt that they could have coped at home with extra help. Overall they report that, while approximately two-thirds of entrants to care had not positively opted for care and were rather resigned to it, they then had participated to some degree in the rest of the process. However, in many cases the admission to care was rapid and there were only limited opportunities for the exercise of choice and the exploration of 'caring options and alternatives' envisaged by the White Paper.

HOW MUCH DO WE SPEND ON LONG-STAY CARE?

The prime motivating force behind the community care changes was the rapid growth in expenditure on long-stay care from the social security budget. It is by now well documented that changes in the rules for the payment of supplementary benefit (now income support), a means-tested benefit for those with very low incomes, meant that 'board and lodging' allowances were paid to those who were unable to afford private or voluntary residential/nursing home care and who the local authority would not support. Laing (1993) argues that one of the main stimuli towards this change was the unwillingness or inability of local authorities to support people in voluntary residential care because of restrictions on their finances. To support this he reports that, in 1974, local authorities paid for 60% of places in voluntary residential homes. By 1983 this had declined to 34%. It is important to note that benefit was not payable to those in local authority run homes, those in NHS long-stay care or to those who wished to remain in their own homes. The only assessment of need made of individuals claiming this benefit was of their financial circumstances. Claimants did not have to demonstrate that their level of frailty meant that they needed long-term care. This system remained in place until the implementation of the community care reforms. However, as time progressed, the benefits became less generous and the criteria for the award more stringent as central government attempted to control the essentially unplanned growth of expenditure in this area.

Laing (1993) argues that it was the voluntary residential homes sector which had argued for this change in benefit rules. However as we saw earlier the major expansion in residential care (and later nursing care) has taken place within the private sector. We saw the tremendous growth in places provided by private operators within the long-stay care market. Table 7.9 indicates the equally, if not more, spectacular growth in social security expenditure used for the support of individuals in long-stay care. We have already highlighted some of the effects resulting from this expenditure. This included the 'perverse' incentive against care at home for individuals who could get help to go into care but not to remain at home. However this perverse incentive also operated at an organizational level. Both the NHS and local authorities were encouraged by the existence of these monies to transfer long-stay care users from their own cash limited budgets into private or voluntary homes where they could receive income support. This change is reflected in the fact that 28% of elderly people in long-stay care in 1970 were receiving 'free' NHS care as compared with 12% in 1992, and 10% in 1996 (Laing, 1993; House of Commons Select Committee on Health, 1996). It is unlikely that the pattern of decreased involvement of the NHS in long-term care will be reversed and that there will be further attempts at 'cost shunting' by redefining health care needs as social care needs.

Laing (1993) has estimated the annual expenditure on long-stay care in the UK. This is shown for older people in Table 7.10. He estimates total expenditure on long-term care for older people at £6612 million a year. This represents 73% of national expenditure in this area. Of this, 23% is funded by the NHS, 12% by local authorities, 30% from social security and the remainder from individuals.

Table 7.9 Income support: recipients in private nursing and
residential homes: Great Britain, 1979–1991[a]

Date		Total recipients	Estimated annual expenditure (£M)
December	1979	11 000	10
	1980	13 000	18
	1981	13 000	23
	1982	16 000	39
	1983	26 000	104
	1984	42 000	200
	1985	70 000	348
February	1986	90 000	459
May	1987	117 000	671
November	1987	131 000	772
May	1988	147 000	878
November	1988	155 000	958
May	1990	189 000	1270
May	1991	231 000	1870
November	1991	252 000	2400

[a]Derived from: Laing, 1993, Table 1

Table 7.10 Estimated expenditure (£m) on long-stay care for older people: UK, 1992[a]

	All ages	Aged 65+	Total (%) those aged 65+
NHS	1716	1550	90
Net local authority	873	807	92
Income support	2143	2009	94
Total net state expenditure	4732	4366	92
User charges	342	319	93
Individual fees	2059	1927	94
Total	7136	6612	93

[a]Derived from: Laing, 1993, Table 3

Although responsible for the lowest percentage, we should not overlook the
significant contribution towards long-stay care being made by older people and
their families. This has become a major social policy and political issue because
of the means-testing of local authority funded long-stay care and the recent debate
about the development of long-term care insurance. However the viability of such
a system is questionable given the low incomes of older people. Although owner
occupation is increasing among older people, Hamnett (1995) estimates that, at
best, 40% of entrants to care would have a property to sell. However the amount
of money required to fund care is significant. If we assume care fees of £300 a
week; with an average stay this would suggest an 'average' bill of £36 000. This
is not an inconsiderable sum and one that is out of reach of the majority of older
people.

The increased importance of the income support system in supporting elderly people in private and voluntary homes is shown in Table 7.11. In 1986 46% of residents of private and voluntary homes paid for themselves and 48% had all (or some) of their fees paid by social security. In 1992 these percentages were 26% and 70% respectively.

Table 7.11 Source of finance for residents in private and voluntary care homes for older people (%), 1986–1992[a]

	1986	1992
Private payers	46	26
Income support (part or all fees)	48	70
Local authority	5	4

[a]Derived from: Laing, 1993, Table 4

This withdrawal of the NHS from long-term care is reflected in their relatively minor importance in the funding of these places. Looking at the institutional responsibility for funding nursing home payments, the ACC/AMA survey (1995) reports that for 75% of placements the local authority would be the main funding body compared with only 9% for the NHS. Only for the London boroughs was there any significant involvement by the NHS in funding nursing home care where 25% of placements were NHS funded and 22% were jointly funded.

There are very marked variations in the amount of money local authorities expect to have to pay for residential and nursing home care costs. For example, 85% of metropolitan districts and 75% of shire counties expect to make nursing home placements for less than £240 per week compared with only 12% of London Boroughs (ACC/AMA, 1995). Similar differentials are evident for residential care.

THE EXPERIENCE OF LONG-STAY CARE

There have been a whole series of reports that have drawn attention to the poor quality of life experienced by older people resident in institutions (Townsend, 1964; Robb, 1967; Meacher, 1972). These authors have all offered incisive critiques of the quality of life and regimens experienced by old people in care. Typical of the observations included within these studies were the dehumanizing nature of the regimens, the lack of choice experienced by residents and the almost total lack of control experienced by older people over their own care. These regimens have been described by Goffman (1968) as characterizing 'the total institution'. This is characterized by three features: all aspects of life are carried out in the same place and under the same authority; each person's life is carried out alongside others who are all treated alike and subject to exactly the same conditions; the daily life of the individual is controlled by a system of formal rules and regulations.

These arguments are well rehearsed and various studies have identified many of the problems that living in an institutional setting can create. However there is now some evidence emerging that conditions are improving and that homes of all varieties have tried to maximize the choice available to residents. For example, Allen *et al*. (1992b) observe that three quarter of the residents they surveyed were satisfied with their home. Positive comments about residential homes often relate to the freedom from worry and the security that such environments can offer. For example 'you get looked after. It's the first rest I've had in years. It's care, attention and kindness ...' (resident of a residential home quoted in Allen *et al*., 1992, p. 199). Similarly a long-stay NHS patient remarked 'we've got no worries, no bills' another stated that not being a burden on the family was important (Higgs *et al*., 1992, p. 291). These statements suggest that there are some positive as well as negative aspects to living in a communal establishment. Considerable improvements have been made in the quality of care offered; although we should not become complacent about this.

Higgs *et al*. (1992) have noted the importance of dependence among the long-stay hospital and nursing home populations which they researched. Overall, residents of long-stay care exhibit high levels of disability and dependence. Many of the negative comments made by older people stem from their forced dependence rather than from the living environment *per se*. It is very difficult, with the best will in the world, for a physically and mentally disabled person to exert much control and choice over their lives. As a consequence we need to guard against the reproduction of many of the features of the 'total institution'; lack of control over daily life, living by timetables set for the convenience of others, and ensure that these are not reproduced in the community when we are developing and implementing complex packages of care for frail people.

ATTITUDES TOWARDS LONG-STAY CARE

In this section we will consider the general attitudes and views of older people and carers towards the different types of long-stay care.

The attitudes of older people

How do older people view the prospect of admission to long-stay care? It is often assumed that older people are strongly opposed to entering residential or NHS/nursing home care. Is this assumption supported by the research evidence? To answer this question fully we need to distinguish between the different types of long-stay care.

Qureshi and Walker (1989) report that in their sample of older people in Sheffield, 40% rejected the idea of residential care, while a further 30% reported that they would only accept admission as a matter of last resort. These responses seem to support the observations of Allen *et al*. (1992b). However, they also report that 3% reported a positive desire to enter residential care while 18% would go 'if necessary'. So, although there is significant opposition to this form of care among older people, it is by no means universal. We must also consider how stable this attitude will be over time. Is the rather negative evaluation of long-term care a feature that is unique to this generation (or cohort) of elders? Will long-stay care be evaluated more positively by future generations of elders?

Qureshi and Walker (1989) looked at the relationship between the importance older people attached to 'independence' and attitudes towards residential care. They report that over 70% of those who rejected the idea of residential care stated that 'independence' was very important to them, compared with 59% who would accept residential care and 50% who were completely willing to enter residential care. However they note that the relationship between independence and residential care is not straightforward. They postulate that for some older people entry into residential care was seen as a way of promoting 'independence' for it meant that they would not have to become dependent upon their children.

Attitudes of older people towards long-stay NHS care is less well researched as are their views about nursing homes. In their Sheffield study, Qureshi and Walker (1989) conclude that attitudes towards geriatric wards were much more negative than those towards residential care. In the Sheffield study the most negatively evaluated dimension of long-stay geriatric care were the number of residents with confusion.

The views of carers

The considerable contribution towards community care made by informal carers has been described. How do they perceive long-stay care? In their survey of 58 carers in Sheffield, Qureshi and Walker (1989) report that 57% totally rejected the idea of residential care; 21% were ambivalent and 10% would accept it if necessary.

What reasons underlay this extensive hostility towards the very idea of long-stay care? Qureshi and Walker (1989) argue that two main factors underpin this belief; the idea that residential care was unacceptable to the older people themselves and the belief that children should, if at all possible, provide the care their parents needed. The unacceptability of residential care to the older person was mentioned by seven out of ten carers in Sheffield. This attitude is exemplified by comments such as 'It's the one thing she is definite about'. 'She doesn't want to go into a home, so that's out. I don't think I'd ever do that, she's always said never put me in a home' (Qureshi and Walker, 1989, p. 197). Furthermore, about half of the carers surveyed felt they could not accept the possibility of entry into residential care because it was up to them to provide whatever was required. As one carer said '... I suppose you must feel you are letting them down in some way', while another reported 'I don't want that on my conscience' (Qureshi and Walker, 1989, p. 197).

However, as Allen et al. (1992b) report many carers are instrumental in the admission of their older relative to care and eventually become quite positive about it. Of the carers they surveyed, over 90% were satisfied with the home and over 50% said their views had changed and that they now had a more positive view. For example 'She is living better than she was before. She has good food regularly and company most of the time' and 'I'd heard some awful stories of the way homes were run but this home is so good. I now realize that residential homes can be marvellous' (Allen *et al.*, 1992, p. 203).

In the Sheffield study there was one aspect of both residential and long-stay care which was of concern, especially to the carers. This was the number of confused residents. One carer described her mother's reaction after visiting an even older relative in a geriatric psychiatry ward as 'Oh don't ever let me come in a place like this, shoot me first, don't ever let me come here' (Qureshi and Walker, 1989, p. 200). Another carer commented after visiting a geriatric ward 'When I saw the people – there was a man walking about wetting himself and a woman sort of [making a wailing noise] all the time – my father wasn't like that and I couldn't have left him' (Qureshi and Walker, 1989, p. 199).

Given these strong views about the number of confused residents, it is one of the ironies of the Sheffield research that carers identified the loss of their dependents mental faculties as the point at which they would consider admission to care. As one daughter said 'I wouldn't like her to go into a home, not as long as she knew what was happening to her'. However, it is clearly seen as acceptable to place people into care when they have become confused. This accords with some general population research which has reported that the appropriate place to care for the confused older person is the institutional/long-stay care sector (West *et al.*, 1984; Victor, 1991).

CONCLUSION

The topic of the role of long-stay care for older people and its role within community care is an extensive one. One of the key issues characteristic of the last decade has been the 'privatization' of long-term care. Much of the supply is now provided by the private sector. However it seems unrealistic to expect current and future generations to be able to pay for such care. As we have seen, the assumption, deriving from 1945, that it is possible to distinguish the sick from the frail continues to be problematic. Defining the boundary between health and social care will, no doubt, continue to be problematic. However, while the debate about who should be cared for by whom continues, there remains a group of frail older people who continue to need care. It is worth reiterating that those in long-stay care represent the largest disability group within the population. They represent very high levels of dependency and often do not have a 'caring network' available to them. Our problem is to find an appropriate and effective model of care which will respond to their needs. With all the focus of attention upon the 'negative' effects of dwelling in an institutional environment it is important to note that many of the features of the total institution can be reproduced by caring for a very dependent person in their own home.

8

Prospects and issues in the development of community care for older people

INTRODUCTION

It is too early to state with any confidence that community care for older people is working. It is too soon after the implementation of this major policy change to come to a definite conclusion. We need longer term data about the quality and quantity of services available and how they do (or do not) respond to users needs before we can pronounce judgement. Several challenges must be faced. If admissions to institutions are to be reduced then we must develop realistic care packages which can support vulnerable people. Can this be achieved under a market system. Can different agencies develop collaborative working required to make these care packages happen. How are we to involve carers? How will expenditure be controlled? Will rationing become more overt? These are just a few of the challenges underpinning the successful implementation of community care. Rather than speculate upon what the answers to these may be, we will consider some of the key issues underlying the future development of community care for older people such as the future of family care and the funding of long-term care. We will conclude by placing the community care debate within a European context. This will indicate that the changes and problems being examined in the UK are not unique to us but are part of a European pattern of social change.

THE PROVISION OF INFORMAL CARE: AN HISTORICAL PERSPECTIVE

One factor which is a key to the success (or otherwise) of community care is the contribution of informal care. One of the issues underlying the development of the post-war welfare state was the very limited degree of domiciliary care provision. It was suggested that this partly reflected the very limited views of those developing policy (they could not imagine that frail older people could be cared for anywhere other than an institution) and partly because they were afraid of undermining the family. Where domiciliary services were being developed, such as the mobile meals service, they were seen as second best to long-stay care and only for the frail living alone; not as a replacement or substitute for the care provided by family members. For example Means and Smith (1985, p. 244) provide a flavour of the feeling on this issue with the following quotation 'if once it were fashionable to transfer the care of the elderly from the family to the state without loss of face and without a guilty conscience, a very big ... problem would confront the community'. It was left to researchers such as Sheldon (1948) and Townsend (1957) to document carefully the powerful contribution which family members were making to the care of older people in the community.

We have carefully documented the invaluable contribution which the family makes to the care of older people in late twentieth century Britain, 35 years after the surveys of Sheldon and Townsend. However, we are still left with an interesting questions – has the contribution of the family increased (or decreased) over this period, in response to the development of state welfare services? This is clearly a difficult problem to solve. To answer this we could compare the results of those obtained by Townsend and Sheldon with those from more recent surveys such as the GHS. However there are difficulties with this approach because no two surveys concerned with informal care ask exactly comparable questions. Given this considerable caveat Table 8.1 compares information from a survey by Townsend and Wedderburn (1965) with data from the 1985 GHS and Sheffield survey of Quershi and Walker (1989). Several trends are evident from this table. First, for the three activities shown; heavy housework, shopping and help with meals, the family has remained the main source of help across the decades. For example, in the Townsend and Wedderburn survey, 80% of people needing help with shopping got this from their family, compared with 68% in the 1985 GHS. For housework the comparable percentages were 69% and 55% respectively, and 83% and 79% for meals. Second, while the contribution made by state services has increased these remain a fairly minimal source of help with the exception of help with housework in the Sheffield survey which reflects the way the sample was chosen. From this albeit limited evidence, we can conclude that the family has remained the main source of help for older people and that there is little evidence that this position has been undermined by the development of state welfare services. Given the stability in the family as a source of informal care across three decades should we assume that things will change radically in the future?

ATTITUDES TOWARDS BECOMING A CARER

As we have already seen in previous chapters, the provision of informal care is a key element in the maintenance of older people (and indeed other care groups) in the community. The lack of an informal carer was a key factor in the entry of older people into institutional care. However, we know relatively little about the willingness (or otherwise) of future generations to take on this role. As we saw earlier, carers are most likely to be drawn from the closest family members (usually a spouse or child). In the future, family relationships are likely to become much more complex, with the increase in divorce and remarriage rates, and it is not clear what effect this will have. Will 'second wives/husbands' feel the same marital obligations as those spouses who have remained married for many decades. Answers to these types of questions will set the framework for the provision of informal care.

Table 8.1 Sources of help for older people: a comparison of studies

	Percentage helped by	
	Townsend and Wedderburn (1965)	Victor (1991)
a) Help with shopping		
Spouse	30	34
Other household member	29	16
Other family member	20	18
Friend/neighbour	10	8
Social services	2	7
Private help	2	1
Other	7	16
b) Heavy housework		
	Townsend and Wedderburn (1965)	Quershi and Walker (1989)
Family	69	55
Friend/neighbour	3	4
Voluntary services	–	1
Social services	9	27
Private	12	–
Other	7	15
c) Meals		
	Townsend and Wedderburn (1965)	Quershi and Walker (1989)
Family	84	79
Friend/neighbour	6	4
Volunteers	–	6
Social services	1	6
Private	2	4
Other	8	–

What do we know about general attitudes towards caring? The CNA (1996) survey is one of the few sources of data investigating general attitudes towards taking on the role of informal carer. Interpretation of the results from this study must be undertaken cautiously as many of the questions posed to respondents were necessarily hypothetical (a cardinal sin in survey research but one perpetrated by many researchers/market researchers – e.g. 'if there was an election tomorrow who would you vote for?'). Overall, 63% of respondents reported that they would willingly become a carer if one of their relatives became frail or disabled (57% of men and 68% of women). In contrast 15% thought they would only do this if there was no alternative and 9% would not do so at all. No difference in responses to these questions were reported with age.

We saw that many carers just grew into that role. It seemed to be a 'natural' development of 'normal' family/marital responsibilities. Certainly the CNA survey suggests that few people think about the possibility of becoming a carer in advance of the event. They report that 54% of people they interviewed had not thought what would happen if a relative/friend could no longer care for themselves. Not surprisingly men were less likely to think about this than women (62% and 47% respectively) and the young (those aged 16–24 years) were least likely (71%) to have contemplated this possibility.

Respondents were then asked about their willingness to care for particular types of people ranging from close relatives to friends/neighbours. The responses to the question are shown in Table 8.2 and these very closely reflect the hierarchy of obligations described by Finch (1989). Three-quarter of respondents were willing to look after a close relative (spouse, parents or dependent child) while only 20% would be prepared to care for non-relatives. The strength of blood ties is highlighted in that 59% of respondents expressed willingness to look after distant relatives compared to 22% for in-laws (this of course may reflect emotional or physical distance or the inclusion within the sample of people who do not have parents in-law). There is little evidence that people would be willing to look after neighbours. This, like the data presented (Chapter 6) confirms that the provision of informal care takes place within the family and rarely ventures beyond its limits. Developing a policy which expects that people will be busy providing care for neighbours, with whom they have not developed reciprocal relationships over a long period of time is clearly doomed to failure.

Table 8.2 Who would you be prepared to look after if they could no longer look after themselves (%)?[a]

	Male	Female	All
Spouse	59	55	57
Parent	55	58	56
Parent in law	21	23	22
Dependent child	33	40	36
Adult child			
Sibling/other	34	38	36
Friend	17	21	19
Neighbour	6	13	9

[a]Derived from: CNA, 1996, Table 6

What kinds of tasks would potential future carers be prepared to undertake? The majority of people surveyed were prepared to undertake help with domestic tasks (shopping, house cleaning, gardening) and personal care tasks such as washing (Table 8.3). Furthermore a substantial percentage of respondents were prepared to give up hobbies (44%), 50% were prepared to change their living arrangements (e.g. sell the house, move in with relative, have relative move in) and one-third (32%) were prepared to make a major job change (give up job or change job). These data suggest that there is an extensive potential pool of carers available to help future generations of elders and certainly does not provide evidence of any significant inter-generation conflict or reluctance to undertake a considerable caring responsibility.

Table 8.3 Which tasks would you undertake to look after friend/relative (%)[a]

	Male	Female	%
Shopping	86	88	87
Spend time with	80	85	82
Household cleaning/gardening	78	80	79
Prepare meals	71	81	76
Take to lavatory	59	74	66
Wash/bath	55	73	64
Change living arrangements	44	56	50
Give up holidays	35	42	39

[a]Derived from: CNA, 1996, Table 7

WHO SHOULD CARE?

We indicated that there was some support for the role of the state in providing care for people with long-term care needs (Chapter 7). Victor (1991) reports that institutional care was seen as being appropriate for those with severe dementia. The sample interviewed in that survey thought it unreasonable that the family should be expected to care for such people. Clearly the general population have a view (possibly misguided and prejudiced) as to who should be cared for at home. This survey also indicates that the population have an expectation that there will be state services to care for people in need. This is an expectation which has developed as a result of the development of a state welfare system which, in theory at least, was to provide a safety net 'from the cradle to the grave'. What do we know about the expectation people have for care in the future and who do they think should provide it?

Providing for the future: expectations of care

According to the CNA (1996) survey, prior to being interviewed 46% of respondents had thought about what they would do if a relative/friend became frail or disabled (38% of males and 53% of females). One third (39%) of the general population had thought about who would care for them if they could not manage because of illness, age or disability (32% of males and 45% of females) compared with 41% of carers. However this percentage does increase with age from 24% of those aged 16–24 years to 55% of those aged 65 years and over (CNA, 1996). It is quite clear that people would expect to receive help from the family if they needed care long-term (Table 8.4). Interestingly it is the young (those aged 16–34 years) who have the highest expectation of receiving care from friends and family. There is little difference in the responses to this question between carers and non-carers. Perhaps older people have a more realistic expectation of the very limited role that the state now plays in the care of people with long-term needs.

Table 8.4 Who would you expect to look after you long term (%)?[a]

	Non carers	Carers
Friends/relatives	63	64
NHS	15	8
Local authority	9	16
Private services	6	7
Other	1	0
Don't know	6	5

[a]Derived from: CNA, 1996

Table 8.5 Who do you think should pay for long term care (%)?[a]

	Non carers	Carers
Central government	45	42
State and family	28	25
Local authority	17	24
Families	3	3
Person concerned	1	1
Other	1	2
Don't know	3	2

[a]Derived from: CNA, 1996

There is an interesting policy issue hinted at in the responses contained in Tables 8.4 and 8.5 Overall, respondents thought that the funding of care for the frail and disabled was a government responsibility. However few of these respondents expected to receive state care; they thought their family would care for them. Clearly these two views are describing different aspects of the population's views about care; perhaps they imply that carers should receive payment for their contribution.

PAYING FOR LONG-TERM CARE

Who does the general population feel should be responsible for paying for the care of frail or disabled adults? Table 8.4 shows that half of both carers and non-carers alike feel that central government should accept financial responsibility for the care of these groups. There is a clear expectation that the welfare state should cover long-term care provision as well as more acute crisis response services. However this expectation is clearly contrary to central government thinking which has been busily trying to divest itself of the financial responsibility for long-term care. One of the reasons why there has been concern about long-term care is the cost and the potential future cost resulting from the 'ageing' of the population.

Providing long-term care: the demographic timebomb?

The overriding question from the government perspective is the cost of long-term care and how this will escalate with the ageing of the British population. As we shall see later in this chapter this is not a demographic feature that is unique to Britain but is a feature of the European situation. It is estimated that 1% of GDP is accounted for by public expenditure on long-term care (Laing, 1993) and that if current tends are forward projected this will rise to 2.5% by 2051. This is then proposed as an unacceptable burden to place upon future generations of workers. However it is important to note that these estimates are based upon lots of assumptions about future patterns of disability/dependence and the availability of informal care. Only time will tell if these were valid. What is important, when evaluating evidence about these issues, is that the assumptions underlying these calculations are examined carefully.

However before we can really undertake such speculative actuarial calculations we need to answer four main questions:

- how will the age composition of the elderly population change in future decades;
- what will be the health status of older people in the future;
- will families in the future be willing to provide informal care and if so to what degree;
- will the cost of providing different types of long-term care change over time.

We cannot answer any of these questions with any degree of precision. Consequently calculations like Laing's above are based upon a set of assumptions which may (or may not) prove to be incorrect. The DoH is much less pessimistic than Laing (1993) and conclude that expenditure may increase to 2% of GDP by 2030 and that this is affordable. Answers to the four questions posed above will help us to answer the questions about the cost of long-term care and by how much this may increase in the future.

There is some support in general population surveys for the idea that long-term care should be funded out of general taxation. Overall 57% of those surveyed in the UK support this idea as compared with 34% in the EC generally (House of Commons Select Committee on Health, 1996). This supports the point noted above that the population of Britain favour a collective rather than individual approach towards the provision of long-stay care. Surveys consistently report that the general population would be willing to pay more in direct taxes to support long-term care for older people. However the evidence from the voting behaviour of the British electorate does not support the answers generated by these hypothetical questions. Nonetheless we may conclude that there is an expectation among the general population that long-term care provision will remain a feature of the welfare state provision in Britain.

Individual provision for long-term care requirements

Laing (1993) estimates total state expenditure on long term care, both in the community and institutions at £7132 million per annum, of which 93% is spent upon older people. In addition older people (or their families) spend a further £2779 million; unpaid informal care is costed at about £32 500 million per annum. For an average older person the cost of long-stay care is estimated at £40 000. This is a significant sum which, it has been suggested, could be covered by some kind of insurance scheme or that older people could meet this out of income or assets.

However, given the very high prevalence of poverty among this segment of the population, this is not a very realistic policy objective. It is estimated that only 4% of people aged 75 years and over, or those in the top 20% of the income distribution, could afford the fees for private care out of income (House of Commons Select Committee on Health, 1996). Some older people, while they might be income poor, can be asset rich in that they own their own home. However it is not clear how realistic an aim this is. A number of insurance companies have developed long-term care insurance. However these are not widely used as the premiums are very expensive. Also, because people feel insecure about the employment market they do not have the confidence to maintain the premiums. Few people have budgeted for long-term care in their later life or made financial planning. It is an assumption by those of middle-age onwards that long-term care in later life is something the state would provide. It is difficult to change the rules of social welfare provision when many potential service users will not be able to alter their financial planning. Certainly the House of Commons Select Committee on Health (1996) do not see a pressing need to change the current system. If any changes were introduced it should be as a result of all party consensus and a thorough review of all aspects of long-term care provision.

The sales of long-term care insurance schemes are extremely limited. This is confirmed by evidence from the 1996 CNA survey. They report that 23% of the population and 16% of carers reported that they had made provision for their future care. However, when asked to identify what arrangements they had made, most were general financial plans such as pensions rather than specific long-term care plans. Hence there is little awareness of or use of long-term care insurance schemes.

THE EUROPEAN PERSPECTIVE ON COMMUNITY CARE

It is not possible to do justice to the complexity of issues encompassed within the title 'European perspectives on community care'. All we can do here is raise some of the pertinent issues. Interested readers are referred elsewhere (Tester, 1996; Jamieson, 1991). Here we will confine our attention to four main topic areas; demography, household composition and family care, and state services both domiciliary services and institutional care.

Population change in Europe

It is easy from the ethnocentric British perspective to assume that population ageing is a feature unique to Britain. This is incorrect. As Table 8.6 shows, Great Britain and Denmark have the highest percentage of their population aged 65 years and over (16%). However, this will not be the case by the year 2000 when this will be Belgium, Germany and Greece. Over the next decade there will be a modest increase (2%) in the percentage aged 65 years and over in Britain, unlike many other European countries where the increase will be 4% or more. Hence, rather than being a time of unique and destabilizing population change, the British population will show little variation in overall composition unlike some of their European contemporaries. This just serves to confirm that population ageing is a factor common to Europe.

Table 8.6 Demographic change in Europe[a]

		% aged 65+		% change	% 65+ living alone
	1975	1990	2000	1975–2000	
Belgium	13	15	17	4	32
Denmark	13	16	16	3	38
Germany	15	15	17	2	39
Greece	12	12	17	5	15
Netherlands	12	13	14	2	36
France	14	14	16	2	32
Spain	11	13	15	4	14
Ireland	10	11	11	1	20
Italy	12	14	16	4	29
Luxembourg	13	14	15	2	23
Portugal	11	13	13	2	18
UK	14	16	16	2	37

[a]Derived from: CPA, 1996, Tables A1 and A2; Tester, 1996, Table 3.1

Household composition and family care

The household composition of older people does show considerable variation across Europe. The prevalence of solo living is highest in the countries of northern Europe and lowest in southern Europe (Table 8.6). There is some evidence that the prevalence of solo living is increasing across Europe. However, regardless of the specific type of household in which European elders live, Jamieson (1991) reports that the main source of care remains the family and that state services, where they exist, complement rather replace family care.

The future supply of family care across Europe will depend upon the inter-relationship between several factors. These include fertility rates, employment rates, marriage rates, divorce rates, migration and remarriage. Clearly we can only speculate as to how these will change across Europe. However it does seem certain that fertility will continue to decline and divorce rates increase. The future families for older people appear to be more complex that todays rather straightforward pattern and that there are likely to be more older people living alone.

In Britain we have seen that family care is very strong and has shown little signs of withering in the face of the development of state community care services. However Salvage (1995) shows that across Europe there is a strong commitment to the ideology of family care for older people, a reluctance to use institutional care and a reluctance to seek statutory help. Salvage suggests we can divide the countries of Europe into three ideological groups with regard to the concept of informal care. These are:

● the replacement of informal care by the state (e.g. Denmark);
● support for carers (e.g. the UK or Netherlands;
● provide a 'safety net' for those without an informal network.

She also notes that across Europe more action is required to develop family care and ensure that it still as vibrant in future decades.

State services for older people

Given the complexity of the organization of formal services for community care (or home care as it is normally termed outside the UK) it is difficult to summarize the varying levels of provision as these reflect the different systems operating in the differing countries. Across Europe the majority of older people (95%) live at home, rates of institutional care provision are reasonably similar across Europe (Table 8.7) as are the levels of domiciliary help provided. Nowhere does the contribution of formal services approach the level of help provided by the informal sector.

Table 8.7 Provision of care in selected European countries[a]

| | Percentage 65+ receiving care | | |
	Long–stay	Home help	Home nursing
France	7.5	3–6	0.6
Germany	7.7	2	3
Italy	2.3	1	–
Netherlands	12.3	8	15
UK	5.7	9	5

[a]Derived from: Tester, 1996, Tables 3.2 and 4.4

CONCLUSION

Hence, across Europe, we can see many similar trends; a desire to reduce the use of institutional care, increased emphasis on home care, an emphasis upon developing social care markets, a stress upon collaboration in care and the development of a concern with the issues of service quality, user choice and empowerment. These are precisely the challenges which face us in the UK. Community care for older people is clearly a social objective with which few would quarrel and it is one with which there is consensus across Europe. However if we are to transform this 'apple pie' statement into a concrete policy which brings worthwhile outcomes to users and carers these challenges have to be overcome.

Bibliography

Allen. I., Dalley, G. and Leat, D. (1992a) *Monitoring change in social services departments*, Policy Studies Institute, London.

Allen, I., Hogg, D and Peace, S, (1992b) *Elderly people: choice, participation and satisfaction*, Policy Studies Institute, London.

Arber, S and Gilbert, N. (1989) Men: the forgotten carers. *Sociology*, 23 (1), 111–118.

Arber, S. and Ginn, J. (1990) The meaning of informal care: gender and the contribution of the elderly. *Ageing and Society*, **10**(4), 429–454.

Arber, S. and Ginn, J. (1991) *Gender and Later Life*, Sage, London.

Arber, S. and Ginn, J. (1995) Gender differences in informal caring. *Health and social care in the community*, **3**, 19–31.

Askham, J. (1995) The married lives of older people, in *Connecting gender and Ageing*, (eds S. Arber J. and Ginn) Open University Press, Milton Keynes, pp. 69–86.

Association of County Councils, Association of Metropolitan Authorities (ACC/AMA) (1995) *Who gets community care?*, AMA, London.

Audit Commission (1986) *Making a reality of community care*, HMSO, London.

Audit Commission (1992) *Managing the cascade of change*, HMSO, London.

Baggott, R. (1994) *Health and social care in Britain*, Macmillan, Basingstoke.

Baldwin, S. (1995) Love and money: the financial consequences of caring for an older relative in *The future of family care for older people*, (eds I. Allen and E. Perkins) HMSO, London pp. 119–140.

Barrett, D. (1993) *Older people, poverty and community care under the Tories*, Avebury, Aldershot.

Barrett, G. and Hudson, M. (1997) Changes in district nursing workload. *Journal of Community Nursing* (in press).

Blakemore, K. and Boneham, M. (1994) *Age, race and ethnicity*, Open University Press, Milton Keynes.

Bowling, A. (1991) *Measuring health: review of quality of life measures*, Open University Press, Milton Keynes.

Bowling, A. (1995) *Measuring disease*, Open University Press, Milton Keynes.

Bowling, A., Farquhar, M. and Grundy, E. (1993) Who are the consistently high users of health and social services? *Health and social care*, **1**, 277–287.

Bradshaw, J. (1972) The concept of social need. *New society*, **30**, 640–643.

Bradshaw, J. and Gibbs, I. (1988) *Public Support for private residential care*, Avebury Gower, Aldershot.

Brayne, C. and Ames, J. (1988) The epidemiology of mental disorders in old age, in *Men-*

tal health in old age, (eds B. Gearing, M. Johnson and T. Heller), Open University Press, Milton Keynes.

Brody, E. (1981) Women in the middle. *The Gerontologist*, **21** (5), 471–479.

Bulmer, M. (1987) *The social basis of community care*, Allen and Unwin, London.

Caldock, K. (1993) A preliminary study of changes in assessment practice – examining the relationship between recent policy and practitioners knowledge and attitudes. *Health and·social care*, **1**, 139–146.

Cambridge, P. (1992) Case management in community services: organizational responses. *British Journal of Social Work*, **22** (5), 495–517.

Carers National Association (CNA) (1992) *Speak up: Speak Out*, CNA, London.

CNA (1996) *Who carers? Perceptions of caring and carers*, CNA, London.

Central Statistical Office (CSO) (1996) *Social trends 1996*, HMSO, London.

Challis, D. and Davies, B. (1986) *Case management in community care: an evaluated experiment in the home care of the elderly*, Gower, Aldershot.

Challis, D., Davies, B. and Trashe, K. (eds) (1994) *Community care: new agencies and challenges from the UK and overseas*, Arena, Aldershot.

Clarke, P. and Bowling, A. (1989) Observation study of quality of life in nursing homes and long-stay wards for the elderly. *Ageing and Society*, **9**, 123–148.

Clifford, D. (1990) *The social costs and rewards of caring*, Avebury, Aldershot.

Dalley, G. (1988) *Ideologies of caring*, Macmillan Education, Basingstoke.

Darton, R. and Wright, K. (1991) Residential and nursing homes for elderly people: one sector or two? in *Elderly people and community care* (eds F. Laczko and C. R. Victor), Avebury, Aldershot, pp. 216–244.

DoH (1996) *Hospital episode statistics; England financial year 1992–3*, DoH, London.

DoH (1989) *Caring for people: community care in the next decade and beyond*, HMSO, London.

DoH (1992) *Implementing caring for people* (Foster-Laming letter), EL92 13/C1/(92)10, DoH, London.

DoH (1993) *Population needs assessment: good practice guide*, DoH, London.

DoH (1995a) *NHS responsibilities for meeting continuing health care needs*, HSG (95)8/LAC (95)5, NHSE, Leeds.

DoH (1995b) *Health and personal social service statistics for England*, HMSO, London.

Department of Health (DoH)/Social services Inspectorate (SSI) (1991a) *Care management and assessment: practitioners guide*, HMSO, London.

DoH/SSI (1991b) *Care management and assessment: managers' guide*, HMSO, London.

DoH/SSI (1991c) *Purchase of service – practice guidance for social services departments and other agencies*, HMSO, London.

DHSS (1978) *A happier old age*, HMSO, London.

DHSS (1981a) *Growing older*, HMSO, London.

DHSS (1981b) *Care in the community. A consultative document on moving resources for care in England*, HMSO, London.

DHSS (1983) *Care in the community and joint finance*, HC (83) 6, DHSS, London.

Ebrahim, S. (1994), Community care – implications for health services for elderly people, in *Community care: new agendas and challenges from the UK and overseas*, (eds D. Challis, B. Davies and K. Tasker), Avebury, Aldershot, pp. 293–303.

Evandrou, M. (1991) Challenging the invisibility of carers: mapping informal care nationally, in *Elderly people and community care*, (eds F. Laczko and C. R. Victor) Avebury, Aldershot, pp. 1–29.

Falkingham J. and Victor, C. R. (1991) The myth of the woopie. *Ageing and Society*, **11** (4), 471–493.

Fell. S. and Foster, A. (1994) *Ages of experience: a survey of attitudes and concerns among older people living in Scotland*, Age Concern, Scotland, Glasgow.

Fennell, G., Phillipson, C. and Evers. H. (1988) *The sociology of old age*, Open University Press, Milton Keynes.

Finch, J. (1989) *Family obligations and social change*, Polity Press, Cambridge.

Finch, J. (1995) Responsibilities, obligations and commitment, in *The future of family care for older people*, (eds I. Allen and E. Perkins), HMSO, London, 51–64.

Finch, J. and Groves, D. (1980) Community care for the elderly: a case for equal opportunities. *Journal of Social Policy*, **9** (4), 487–514.

Finch, J. and Groves, D. (eds) (1983) *A labour of love; women, work and caring*, Routledge and Kegan Paul, London.

Fisher, M. (1990) Defining the practice content of care management. *Social work and social services review*, **2** (3), 204–230.

Fletcher, A. (1994) Properties of assessment instruments in *Assessing elderly people in hospital and community care*, (ed. I. Philp) Farrand Press, London, pp. 25–34.

GHS (1996) *Living in Britain: results form the 1994 GHS*, (eds Bennett, N., Harvis, L., Rolands, D. *et al*.), HMSO, London.

Glendenning, C. and Bewley (1992) *Involving disabled people in community care planning*, Department of Social Policy and Social Work, University of Manchester.

Goddard, E. and Savage, D (1994) *People aged 65 and over*, series GHS 22 supplement A, OPCS, London.

Goffman, E. (1968) *Asylums*, Penguin, Harmondsworth.

Grant, G. and Nolan, M. (1993) Informal carers – sources and concomitant of satisfaction. *Health and social care*, **1**, 147–159.

Green, H. (1988) *Informal carers*, series GHS, 15, supplement A, OPCS, HMSO, London.

Griffiths, R. (1988) *Community care: agenda for action*, HMSO, London.

Groves, D (1995) Costing a fortune: pensioners' financial resources in the context of community care, in *The future of family care for older people*, (eds I. Allen and E. Perkins), HMSO, London, pp. 141–162.

Grundy, E. (1995) Demographic influences on the future of family care, in *The future of family care for older people*, (eds I. Allen I. and E. Perkins), HMSO, London, pp. 1–17.

Ham, C. (1992) *Health policy in Britain*, 3rd edn, Macmillan, Basingstoke.

Hamnet, C. (1995) Housing, equity release and inheritance, in *The future of family care for older people*, (eds I. Allen and E. Perkins), HMSO, London, pp. 163–180.

Hancock, R. and Jarvis, R. (1994) *The long-term effects of being a carer*, HMSO, London.

Hancock, R. and Weir (1994) *More ways than means: a guide to pensioners' incomes*, Age Concern Institute of Gerontology, London.

Henwood, M., Jowell, T. and Wistow, G. (1991) *All things come to those who wait*, King's Fund Institute, London.

Herrington, R. (1996), An analysis of the elderly's comprehensive assessment from all Greater London Boroughs, St George's Hospital Medical School, University of London. Unpublished MSc thesis.

Higgs, P., MacDonald, L. and Ward, M. C. (1992) Responses to the institution among elderly patients in hospital long-stay wards. *Social Science and Medicine*, **35** (3), 287–293.

Hill, M. (1993) *Understanding social policy*, 4th edn, Blackwell, Oxford.

House of Commons Select Committee on Health (1996) *The future and funding of long-term care* (2 vols), HMSO, London.

House of Commons Select Committee on Social Services (1985) Community care volume, report HC 13-1, session 84/85, HMSO, London.

Hoyes, L. and Means, R. (1993) Markets, contracts and social care services: prospects and problems in *Community care; a reader,* (ed. J. Bornat), Macmillan, Basingstoke, pp. 287–295.

Hughes, B. (1995) *Older people and community care,* Open University Press, Milton Keynes.

Hunter, D. and Judge K. (1988) *Griffiths and community care: meeting the challenge,* briefing paper 5, King's Fund, London.

Impallomeni, M. and Starr, J. (1995) The changing face of community and institutional care for the elderly. *Journal of Public Health Medicine,* **17**(2), 171–178.

Jamieson, A. (ed) (1991) *Home care for older people in Europe,* Oxford University Press, Oxford.

Jarvis, C., Hancock, R., Askham, J. and Tinker, A. (1996) *Getting around after 60: a profile of Britain's older population,* Age Concern Institute of Gerontology, London.

Jefferys, M. (1983) The over eighties in Britain: the social construction of a moral panic. *Journal of Public Health Policy,* **4**, 367–372.

Jinkinson, C. (ed.) (1994) *Measuring health and medical outcomes,* UCL Press, London.

Johnson, P. and Falkingham, J. (1992) *Ageing and economic welfare,* Sage, London.

Jorm, A. F., Korten, A. and Hendeson, A. S. (1987) The prevalence of dementia: a quantitative integration of the literature. *Acta Psychiatrica Scandinavia,* **76**, 465–479.

Joshi, H. (1995) The labour market and unpaid caring: conflict and compromise, in *The future of family care for older people,* (eds I. Allen and E. Perkins), HMSO, London, pp. 93–118.

Laczko, F. and Phillipson, C. (1991) *Changing work and retirement,* Open University Press, Milton Keynes.

Laing, W. (1993) *Financing long-term care: the crucial debate.* Age Concern, London.

Land, H. (1978) Who cares for the family? *Journal of Social Policy,* **7** (3), 357–384.

Leicester, M. (1994) Needs assessment for community care in South Thames (West), Faculty of Public Health medicine. Unpublished part two project.

Leicester, M. and Pollock, A. (1996) Community care in South Thames (West) Region – is needs assessment working? *Public Health,* **110**, 109–113.

Leicester, M., Godden, S., Jones, F. and Pollock, A. (1996) *IM. and T. support for care in the community,* Department of Public Health, MSW Health Commission.

Lewis, J. and Meredith, B. (1988) *Daughters who care,* Routledge, London.

Local Government Management Board (LGMB) (1994) *From social security to community care: the impact of the transfer of funding on local authorities,* LGMB, Luton.

LGMB (1996) *Community care trends,* LGMB, Luton.

Marks, L. (1994) *Seamless care or patchwork quilt, discharging patients from acute hospital care,* research report 17, Kings Fund Institute, London.

Martin, J., Meltzer. H. and Elliot, D. (1988) *The prevalence of disability amongst adults,* HMSO, London.

Maxwell, R. J. (1984) Quality Assessment In Health. *British Medical Journal,* **288**, 1470–1473.

McLaughlin, E. and Ritchie, J. (1994) Legacies of caring: the experiences and circumstances of ex-carers. *Health and social care,* **2**, 241– 253.

McWalter, G., Toner, H., Croser, A. *et al.* (1994) Needs and needs assessment: their components and definitions with reference to dementia. *Health and social care,* **2**, 213–219.

Meacher, M. (1972) *Taken for a ride,* Longman, London.

Means, R. and Smith, R. (1985) *The development of welfare services for elderly people*, Croom Helm, Beckenham.

Means, R. and Smith, R.. (1995) *Community care: policy and practice*, Macmillan, Basingstoke.

Meredith, B. (1995) *The community care handbook*, Age Concern, London.

MoH (1957) *Geriatric services on the chronic sick*, HMSO, London.

MoH (1957) *Local authority services for the chronic sick and infirm*, HMSO, London.

MoH (1965) *The care of the elderly in hospitals and residential homes*, HMSO, London.

NHSCCA Act (1990) HMSO, London.

Nissel, M. and Bonnerjea, L. (1982) *Family care of the elderly: who pays?*, Policy Studies Institute, London.

Nolan, M., Grant, G. and Ellis, N. (1990) Stress is in the eye of the beholder. *Journal of Advanced Nursing*, **15**, 544–555.

Norman, A. (1985) *Triple jeopardy*, Centre for Policy on Ageing, London.

OPCS (1992) *Carers in the 1990 GHS*, OPCS monitor ss 92/2, HMSO, London.

OPCS (1995a) *The General Household Survey 1993*, HMSO, London.

OPCS (1995b) *1992 based National Population Projections*, OPCS, HMSO, London.

OPCS (1996) Population and health monitor, DH2 96/2 Deaths by cause, OPCS, London.

Parker, G. (1990) *With due care and attention*, 2nd edn, Family Studies Policy Centre, London.

Parker, G. and Lawton, D. (1994) *Different types of care – different types of carers*, HMSO, London.

Payne, M. (1993) Routes to and through clienthood and their implications for practice. *Practice*, **6**(3), 169–180.

Phillips, J. (1994) The employment consequences of caring for older people. *Health and Social Care*, **2**, 143–152.

Pickin, C. and St Leger, S. (1993) *Assessing health needs across the life cycle*, Open University Press, Milton Keynes.

Price Waterhouse/DoH (1991) *Implementing community care: purchaser, commissioner and provider roles*, HMSO, London.

Qureshi, H. and Walker, A. (1989) *The caring relationship*, Macmillan, Basingstoke.

Robb, B.. (ed.) (1967) *Sans everything*, Nelson, London.

Robins, A. and Wittenberg, R. (1992) The health of elderly people, in, *The health of elderly people: an epidemiological overview*, companion papers to volume 1, HMSO, London.

Rose, H. and Bruce, E. (1995) Mutual care but differential esteem, in *Connecting gender and ageing*, (eds S. Arber and J. Ginn), Open University Press, Milton Keynes, pp. 114–128.

Royal College of Physicians, British Geriatric Society (RCP/BGS) (1992) *Standardised assessment scales for elderly people*, RCP, London.

Salvage, A. (1995) *Who will care?* European Foundation, London.

Scharf, T. and Wenger, C. (eds) (1995) *International perspectives on community care for older people*, Avebury, Aldershot.

Sheldon, J. (1948) *The social medicine of old age*, Oxford University Press, Oxford.

Sinclair, I. (ed.) (1988) *Residential care: the research reviewed*, HMSO, London.

Social Services Inspectorate (SSI) (1994) *Inspection of assessment and care management in social services departments*, second overview report, DoH, London.

Stern, M. C., Jagger, C., Clarke, M. *et al*. (1993) Residential care for elderly people: a decade of change. *British Medical Journal*, **306**, 827–830.

Stevens, A. and Raferty, J. (1994) Introduction, in *Health care needs assessment*, (eds A.

Stevens and J. Raferty), Radcliffe, Oxford.

St Leger, S., Shneiden, H. and Walsworth Bell, J. P. (1992), *Evaluating health services' efficiency*, Open University Press, Milton Keynes.

Tester, S. (1996) *Community care for older people in Europe*, Macmillan, Basingstoke.

Tinker, A., McCreadie, C., Wright, F. and Salvage, A. (1994), *The care of frail elderly people in the United Kingdom*, HMSO, London.

Titmus, R. (1968) *Commitment to welfare*, Allen and Unwin, London.

Townsend, P. (1957) *The family life of old people*, Routledge and Kegan Paul, London.

Townsend, P. (1964) *The last refuge*, Routledge and Kegan Paul, London.

Townsend, P. (1979) *Poverty in the United Kingdom*, Penguin, Harmondsworth.

Townsend, P. (1981) The structured dependency of the elderly: the creation of social policy in the twentieth century. *Ageing and Society*, **1**(1), 5–28.

Townsend, P. and Wedderburn, D. (1965) *The aged in the welfare state*, Bell, London.

Tremellan, J. and Jones, D. A. (1989) Attitudes and practices of the primary health care team towards assessing the very elderly. *Journal of the Royal College of General Practitioners*, **39**, 142–144.

Twigg, J. (ed.) (1992) *Carers: research and practice*, HMSO, London.

Ungerson, C. (1987) *Policy is personal: sex, gender and informal care*, Tavistock, London.

Vetter, N. J., Jones, D. A. and Victor, C. R. (1984) The effectiveness of health visitors working with elderly patients in general practice. *British Medical Journal*, **288**, 369–372.

Victor, C. R. (1987) *Old age in modern society*, 1st edn, Croom Helm, Beckenham.

Victor, C. R. (1990) A survey of the delayed discharge of elderly people from hospital in an inner city health district. *Archives of Gerontology and Geriatrics*, **4**, 117–124.

Victor, C. R. (1991) *Health and health care in later life*, Open University Press, Milton Keynes.

Victor, C. R. (1994) *Old age in modern society*, Chapman and Hall, London (second edition).

Victor, C. R. (1996a) The financial circumstances of older people, in *Developing services for older people and their families*, (ed. R. Bland), Jessica Kingsley, London, pp. 43–57.

Victor, C. R. (1996b) *How useful are health outcome measures with older people?* Paper presented at joint BGS/BSRA/BSG conference, Manchester.

Victor, C. R., Nazareth, B., Hudson, M. and Fulop, N. (1993) The inappropriate use of acute beds in an inner London DHA. *Health Trends*, **25**(3), 94–97.

Warner N. (1994) *Just a fairy tale: carers and community care*, CNA, London.

Wenger, G. C. (1984) *The supportive network*, Allen and Unwin, London.

Wenger, G. C. (1994) *Understanding support networks and community care*, Avebury, Aldershot.

West, P., Illsley, R. and Iselman, M. (1984) Public preference for the care of dependent groups. *Social Science and Medicine*, **18**(4), 417–426.

Williamson, J., Stokoe, I. H., Gray, S. and Fisher, M. (1964) Old people at home – their unreported needs. *Lancet*, **i**, 1117–1120.

Wilson, G. (1994) Assembling their own care packages; payments for care by men and women in advanced old age. *Health and Social Care*, **2**, 283–291.

Wilson, G. (1995) I'm the eyes and she's the arms – changes in gender roles in advanced old age, in *Connecting gender and ageing*, (eds S. Arber and J. Ginn) Open University Press, Milton Keynes, pp. 98–113.

Index